HOW THE
IMMUNE SYSTEM WORKS,
2ND Edition

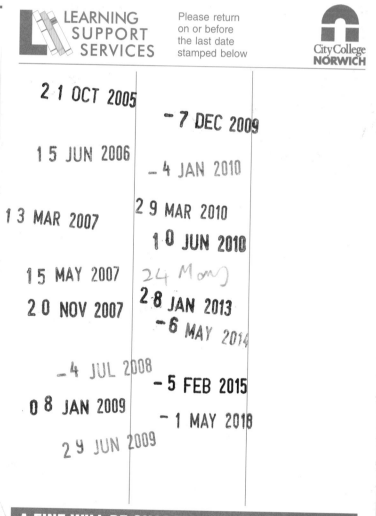

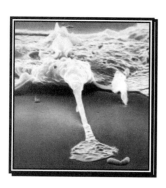

HOW THE IMMUNE SYSTEM WORKS,
2ND Edition

LAUREN SOMPAYRAC, PhD

Retired Professor
Department of Molecular, Cellular, and Developmental Biology
University of Colorado
Boulder, Colorado

Blackwell
Publishing

© 2003 by Blackwell Science
a Blackwell Publishing company

Blackwell Publishing, Inc., 350 Main Street, Malden, Massachusetts 02148-5018, USA
Blackwell Science Ltd, Osney Mead, Oxford OX2 0EL, UK
Blackwell Science Asia Pty Ltd, 550 Swanston Street, Carlton South, Victoria 3053, Australia
Blackwell Verlag GmbH, Kurfürstendamm 57, 10707 Berlin, Germany

02 03 04 05 5 4 3 2 1

ISBN: 0-632-04702-X

Library of Congress Cataloging-in-Publication Data

Sompayrac, Lauren.
    How the immune system works / Lauren Sompayrac. – 2nd ed.
       p.   ;   cm.
    Includes index.
    ISBN 0-632-04702-X
    1. Immune system.   2. Immunity.   I. Title.
    [DNLM: 1. Immune System–physiology.   2. Immune System
–anatomy & histology.   3. Immune System–physiopathology.
    4. Immunity–physiology. QW 504 S697h 2003]
    QR181.S65 2003
    616.07'9–dc21

2002014141

A catalogue record for this title is available from the British Library

Acquisitions: Nancy Anastasi Duffy
Development: Amy Nuttbrock
Production: Debra Lally
Cover design: Meral Dabcovich
Typesetter: SNP Best-set Typesetter Ltd., Hong Kong
Printed and bound by Edwards Bros. in Ann Arbor, MI

For further information on Blackwell Publishing, visit our website:
www.medirect.com

Notice: The indications and dosages of all drugs in this book have been recommended in the medical literature and conform to the practices of the general community. The medications described do not necessarily have specific approval by the Food and Drug Administration for use in the diseases and dosages for which they are recommended. The package insert for each drug should be consulted for use and dosage as approved by the FDA. Because standards for usage change, it is advisable to keep abreast of revised recommendations, particularly those concerning new drugs.

DEDICATION

I dedicate this book to my sweetheart, my best friend, and my wife: Vicki Sompayrac.

ACKNOWLEDGMENTS

I would especially like to thank Dr. Eric Martz, who used the first edition of *How the Immune System Works* in his classes at the University of Massachusetts at Amherst. Many of the improvements in this book result from his thoughtful and detailed critique of the first edition.

I would also like to thank the following people whose critical comments on the first and second editions were most helpful: Drs. Mark Dubin, Linda Clayton, Dan Tenen, Jim Cook, Tom Mitchell, and Lanny Rosenwasser. Thanks also go to Diane Lorenz, who illustrated the first edition, and whose wonderful artwork can still be found in this book. Finally I wish to thank Vicki Sompayrac, whose wise suggestions helped make this book more readable, and whose editing was invaluable in preparing the final manuscript.

CONTENTS

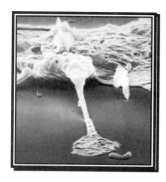

HOW TO USE THIS BOOK

I wrote *How the Immune System Works* because I couldn't find a book that would give my students an overall view of the immune system. Sure, there are as many good, thick textbooks as a person might have money to buy, but these are crammed with every possible detail. There are also lots of "review books" that are great if you want a summary of what you've already learned – but they won't <u>teach</u> you immunology. What was missing was a short book that tells, in simple language, how the immune system fits together – a book that presents the big picture of the immune system, without the jargon and the details.

How the Immune System Works is written in the form of "lectures," because I want to talk to you directly, just as if we were together in a classroom. This book is short, so you should be able to finish it in a few days. In fact, I strongly suggest that you sit down with this little book and read it from start to finish. The whole idea is to get an overall view of the subject, and if you read one lecture a week, that won't happen. Don't "study" this book the first time through – just enjoy it. Later you can go back and reread the appropriate lectures as your immunology course progresses – to keep you from losing sight of the big picture as the details get filled in.

Although the first lecture is a light-hearted overview meant to give you a running start at the subject, you'll soon discover that this is not "baby immunology." *How the Immune System Works* is a concept-driven analysis of <u>how the immune system players work together</u> to protect us from disease – and <u>why</u> they do it this way.

In some settings, *How the Immune System Works* will serve as the main text for the immunology section of a larger course. In a semester-long undergraduate or graduate immunology course, your professor may use this book either as a companion to a detailed text or as the central text, supplemented by additional readings.

No matter how your professor may choose to use this book, however, you should keep one important point in mind: I didn't write *How the Immune System Works* for your professor. This book's for <u>you</u>!

PART I

The Healthy Immune System

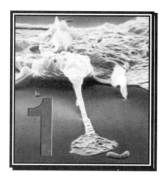

AN OVERVIEW

Immunology is a difficult subject to study for several reasons. First, there are lots of details, and sometimes these details get in the way of understanding the concepts. To get around this difficulty, we're going to concentrate on the big picture – it will be easy for you to find the details somewhere else. A second difficulty in learning immunology is that there is an exception to every rule. Immunologists love these exceptions, because they give clues as to how the immune system functions. But for now, we're just going to learn the rules. Oh, sure, we'll come upon exceptions from time to time, but we won't dwell on them. Our goal will be to examine the immune system, stripped to its essence. The third difficulty in studying immunology is that our knowledge of the immune system is still evolving. As you'll see, there are many unanswered questions, and some of the things that seem true today will be proven false tomorrow. I'll try to give you a feeling for the way things stand now, and from time to time I'll discuss what immunologists speculate may be true. But keep in mind that although I'll try to be straight with you, some of the things I'll tell you will change in the future (maybe even by the time you read this!).

Probably the main reason immunology is such a tough study, however, is that the immune system is really a "network" that involves many different players which interact with each other. Imagine you're watching a football game on TV, and the camera is isolated on one player, say, the tight end. You see him run full speed down the field, and then stop. It doesn't seem to make any sense. Later, however, you see the same play on the big screen, and now you understand: That tight end took two defenders with him down the field, leaving the running back uncovered to catch the pass and run for a touchdown. The immune system is just like a football team. It's a network of players who cooperate to get things done, and just looking at one player doesn't make much sense. You need an overall view. That's the purpose of this first lecture, which you might call "turbo immunology." Here, I'm going to take you on a quick tour of the immune system, so you can get a feeling for how it all fits together. Then in the next lectures, we'll go back and take a closer look at the players and their interactions.

PHYSICAL BARRIERS

Our first line of defense against invaders consists of physical barriers. Although we tend to think of our skin as the main barrier, the area covered by our skin is only about two square meters. In contrast, the area covered by the mucous membranes that line our digestive, respiratory, and reproductive tracts measures about 400 square meters. So there is a large perimeter that must be defended. To cause trouble, viruses, bacteria, and parasites must first get past the physical barriers that protect this perimeter.

THE INNATE IMMUNE SYSTEM

Any invader that breaches the physical barrier of skin or mucosa is greeted by the innate immune system – our second line of defense. Immunologists call this system "innate" because it is a defense that all animals just naturally seem to have. The way the innate system works is pretty amazing.

Imagine you are getting out of your hot tub, and as you step onto the deck, you get a large splinter in your big toe. On that splinter are lots of bacteria, and within a few hours you'll notice (unless you had a lot to drink in that hot tub!) that the area around where the splinter entered is red and swollen – indications that your innate immune system has kicked in. In your tissues are roving bands of white blood cells that defend you against attack. To us, tissue looks pretty solid – that's because we're so big. To a cell, tissue looks somewhat like a sponge with holes through which individual cells can move rather freely. One of the defender cells that is stationed in your tissues is the most famous innate immune system player of them all: the macrophage. If you are a bacterium, a macrophage is the last cell you want to see after your ride on that splinter. Here is an electron micrograph showing a macrophage about to devour a bacterium:

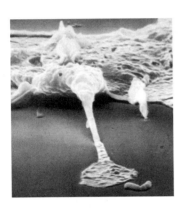

What you'll notice is that the macrophage is not waiting until it bumps into the bacterium. No, it's reaching out to grab it, because bacteria and other invaders give off chemical signals that actually attract macrophages. When it encounters a bacterium, the macrophage first engulfs it in a pouch (vesicle) called a "phagosome." This vesicle is then taken inside the macrophage. There it fuses with another vesicle called a "lysosome," which contains powerful chemicals and enzymes that can destroy the bacterium. This whole process is called "phagocytosis," and this series of snapshots shows how it happens:

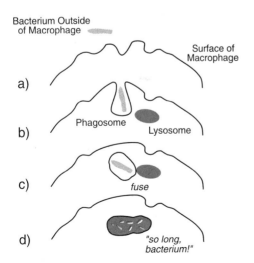

Why is this creature called a macrophage, you may be wondering. "Macro," of course, means large – and a macrophage is a large cell. Phage comes from a Greek word meaning "to eat." So a macrophage is a big eater. In fact, in addition to defending against invaders, the macrophage functions as a garbage collector. It will eat almost anything. Immunologists take advantage of this appetite by feeding macrophages iron filings. Then, using a small magnet, they can separate macrophages from other cells in a cell mixture. Really!

Where do macrophages come from? Macrophages and all the other blood cells in your body are made in the bone marrow where they descend from self-renewing cells called stem cells – the cells from which all the blood cells "stem." By self-renewing, I mean that when a stem cell grows and divides into two daughter cells, it does a "one for me, one for you" thing in which some of the daughter cells go back to being stem cells, and some of the daughters go on to become mature blood cells. As each daughter cell matures, it has to make choices that determine which type of blood cell it will be when it grows up. As you can imagine, these choices are not random, but are carefully controlled to make sure you have enough of each kind of blood cell. Here is a figure showing some of the many different kinds of blood cells (macrophage, neutrophil, red blood cell, etc.) a stem cell can become:

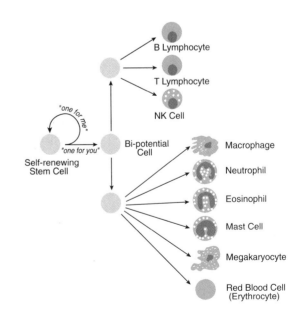

When macrophages first exit the bone marrow and enter the blood stream, they are called monocytes. All in all you have about two billion of these "young macrophages" circulating in your blood at any one time. This may seem a little creepy, but you can be very glad they are there. Without them, you'd be in deep trouble. Monocytes remain in the blood for an average of about three days. During this time they travel to the capillaries, which represent the "end of the line" as far as blood vessels go, looking for a crack between the endothelial cells that line the capillaries. These cells are shaped like shingles, and by sticking a foot between them, the monocyte can leave the blood, enter the tissues, and mature into a macrophage. Once in the tissues, most macrophages just hang out, do their garbage collecting thing, and wait for you to get that splinter so they can do some real work.

When macrophages eat the bacteria on that splinter, they give off chemicals which increase the flow of blood to the vicinity of the wound. The build-up of blood in this area is what makes your toe red. Some of these chemicals cause the cells that line the blood vessels to contract, leaving spaces between them so that fluid in the capillaries can leak into the tissues. It is this fluid that causes the swelling. In addition, chemicals released by macrophages can stimulate nerves in the tissues that surround the splinter, sending pain signals to your brain to alert you that something isn't quite right in the area of your big toe.

During their battle with bacteria, macrophages also produce proteins called cytokines. These are hormone-like messengers that facilitate communication between cells of the immune system. Some of the cytokines alert macrophages and other immune system cells traveling in nearby capillaries that the battle is on, and influence these cells to exit the blood to help fight the rapidly multiplying bacteria. I should also point out that macrophages are not very tidy eaters. They frequently burp some of their meal back out into the tissues, and this debris also serves as a signal to recruit more defenders from the blood. Pretty soon you have a vigorous "inflammatory" response going on in your toe, as the innate immune system battles to eliminate the invaders.

When you think about it, this is a great strategy. You have a large perimeter to defend, so you station sentinels (macrophages) to check for invaders. When these sentinels encounter the enemy, they send out signals that recruit more defenders to the site of the battle. The macrophages then do their best to hold off these invaders until the reinforcements arrive. Because the innate response involves players like macrophages that are programmed to recognize many of the most common invaders, your innate immune system usually responds so quickly that the battle is over in just a few days. Why, by next Saturday night, your toe should be all well and ready for another dip in that hot tub!

There are other players on the innate team, and we will talk about them at length in the next lecture. For example, in addition to cells like macrophages, which make it their business to eat invaders (the so-called "professional phagocytes"), the innate system includes the complement proteins that can punch holes in bacteria, and some rather mysterious cells called natural killer cells. These natural killer cells are able to destroy bacteria, parasites, virus-infected cells, and cancer cells. The mystery is how they know what to kill.

THE ADAPTIVE IMMUNE SYSTEM

About 99% of all animals get along just fine with only natural barriers and the innate immune system to defend them. However, for the vertebrates like us, Mother Nature has laid on a third level of defense: the adaptive immune system. This is a defense system that actually can adapt to protect us against almost any invader.

Opinions vary on why this extra level of protection is needed. Some say it's because vertebrates are more complex or because they have fewer offspring. There are even those who believe that the adaptive immune system was designed to protect us against cancer, but I'm not buying that. Cancer is mostly a disease of old age, and evolutionary pressure to survive decreases after animals have finished bearing and raising their young. So the adaptive system probably didn't evolve to deal with cancer. No, it is most likely that the adaptive immune system was designed to protect us and the other vertebrates against viruses, because as you will see, the innate immune system isn't terribly effective against viruses.

One of the first clues that the adaptive immune system existed came in the 1790s when Edward Jenner began vaccinating the English against smallpox virus. In those days, smallpox was a major health problem. Hundreds of thousands of people died from this disease, and many more were horribly disfigured. What Jenner noticed was that milkmaids frequently contracted a disease called cowpox, which caused lesions on their hands that looked similar to the sores caused by the smallpox virus. Moreover, Jenner noted that milkmaids who had had cowpox almost never got smallpox (which, it turns out, is caused by a close relative of the cowpox virus).

So Jenner decided to do a daring experiment. He collected pus from the sores of a milkmaid who had cowpox, and used this to inoculate a little boy named James Phipps. Later, when Phipps was re-inoculated with pus from the sores of a person infected with small-pox, he did not contract the disease. In Latin, the word for cow is *vacca* – which explains where we get the word vaccine. History makes out the hero in this affair to be Edward Jenner, but I think the real hero that day was the young boy. Imagine having this big man approach you with a large needle and a tube full of pus! Although this isn't the sort of thing that could be done today, we can be thankful that Jenner's experiment was a success, because it paved the way for vaccinations that have saved countless lives.

One important point about this smallpox vaccina-tion is that it only protected against smallpox or closely related viruses like cowpox. Phipps was still able to get mumps, measles, and the rest. This is one of the hall-marks of the adaptive immune system: It adapts to defend against <u>specific</u> invaders.

ANTIBODIES AND B CELLS

Eventually, immunologists determined that im-munity to smallpox was due to special proteins that circulated in the blood of immunized individuals. These proteins were named antibodies, and the agent that caused the antibodies to be made was called the antigen – in this case, the cowpox virus. Here's a sketch that shows the prototype antibody, immunoglobulin G (IgG):

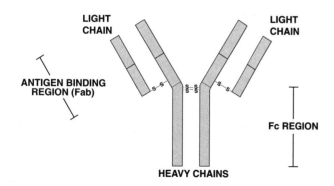

As you can see, an IgG antibody molecule is made up of two pairs of two different proteins, the heavy chain and the light chain. Because of this structure, each molecule has two identical "hands" (Fab regions) that can bind to antigens. IgG makes up about 75% of the antibodies in the blood, but there are four other classes of antibodies: IgA, IgD, IgE, and IgM. All of these anti-bodies are produced by "B cells" – white blood cells that are born in the bone marrow, and which then mature to become antibody factories called "plasma" B cells.

In addition to binding to antigens with its hands, the constant region (Fc) "tail" of the antibody can bind to receptors (Fc receptors) on the surfaces of cells like macrophages. In fact, it is the special structure of the antibody Fc region that determines its class (e.g., IgG vs. IgA), which immune system cells it will bind to, and how it will function.

Each antibody binds to a specific antigen (e.g., a protein on the surface of the smallpox virus), so in order to have antibodies available that can bind to many dif-ferent antigens, many different antibody molecules are required. Now, if we want antibodies to protect us from every possible invader (and we do!), how many differ-ent antibodies would we need? Well, immunologists have made rough estimates that about 100 million should do the trick. Since each antigen binding region of an antibody is composed of a heavy chain and a light chain, we could mix and match about 10,000 different heavy chains and 10,000 different light chains to get the 100 million different antibodies we need. However, human cells have only about 40,000 genes in all, so if each heavy and light chain were encoded by a different gene, about half the cell's genes would be used up just to make antibodies. You see the problem.

GENERATING ANTIBODY DIVERSITY

The solution to the riddle of how B cells produce antibodies with enough different kinds of "hands" to protect us from all invaders actually has two parts. The first is called the principle of clonal selection. The second has to do with the way antibody genes are con-structed – by modular design.

CLONAL SELECTION

The principle of clonal selection holds that each B cell makes antibodies that have only one type of antigen binding region, and which therefore are specific for a certain antigen, called its "cognate" antigen. These antibodies are displayed on the surface of the B cell, and it is through these surface antibodies (called B cell receptors or BCRs) that the B cell is able to know that its cognate antigen is "out there." You see, cells are basically blind to what is going on outside them, so they use antenna-like receptors that span the cell membrane to recognize certain molecules on the outside, and to relay this information to the inside of the cell. In this way, cells are able to sense the environment in which they live and react to it. Each B cell has thousands of BCRs on its surface, but all the receptors on a given B cell recognize the same cognate antigen.

When the B cell receptor binds to its cognate antigen, the B cell is triggered to double in size and divide into two daughter cells – a process immunologists call "proliferation." Both daughter cells then double in size and divide to produce a total of four cells, and so forth. Each cycle of cell growth and division takes about twelve hours to complete, and this period of proliferation usually lasts about a week. At the end of this time, a "clone" of roughly 20,000 identical B cells will have been produced, all of which have receptors on their surfaces that can recognize the same antigen. Most members of this clone will eventually mature into plasma B cells, which will produce and export huge quantities of antibodies into the blood and tissues.

So when a B cell recognizes its cognate antigen, that B cell is <u>selected</u> to proliferate in order to make a clone of B cells, all of which have receptors that recognize the same antigen. This clonal selection principle is recognized as one of the major concepts in immunology.

MODULAR DESIGN

Given that each B cell makes only one kind of antibody, we are still faced with the problem of how to make 100 million different B cells that can be selected, when needed, to produce the antibodies required to protect us. This riddle was finally solved in 1977 by Susumu Tonegawa, who received the Nobel Prize for his discovery. When Tonegawa started working on this problem, the dogma was that the DNA in every cell in the body was the same. This made perfect sense, because after an egg is fertilized, the DNA in the egg is copied. These copies are then passed down to the daughter cells, where they are copied again, and passed down to their daughters, etc. Therefore, barring errors in copying, each of our cells should end up with the same DNA as the fertilized egg. Tonegawa, however,

hypothesized that although this is probably true in general, there might be exceptions. His idea was that all of our B cells might start out with the same DNA, but that as these cells mature, the DNA that makes up the antibody genes might change – and these changes might be enough to generate the 100 million different antibodies we need.

Tonegawa decided to test this hypothesis by comparing the DNA sequence of the light chain from a mature B cell with the DNA sequence of the light chain from an immature B cell. Sure enough, he found they were different, and that they were different in a very interesting way. What Tonegawa and others discovered was that the mature antibody genes are made by modular design!

In every B cell, on the chromosomes that encode the antibody heavy chain, there are multiple copies of four types of DNA modules (gene segments) called V, D, J, and C. Each copy of a given module is slightly different from the other copies of that module. For example, in humans there are about fifty different V segments, about twenty different D segments, six different J segments, etc. To assemble a mature heavy chain gene, each B cell chooses (more or less at random) one of each kind of segment and pastes them together like this:

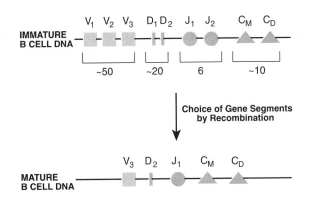

You have seen this kind of mix and match strategy used before to create diversity. For example, twenty different amino acids are mixed and matched to create the huge number of different proteins that our cells produce. And to create genetic diversity, chromosomes you inherited from your mother and father are mixed and matched to make the set of chromosomes that goes into your egg or sperm cells. Once Mother Nature gets a good idea, she uses it over and over – and this modular design idea is one of her very best!

The DNA that encodes the light chain of the antibody molecule is also assembled by picking gene segments and pasting them together. Because there are so many different gene segments that can be mixed and matched, this scheme can be used to create about 10 million different antibodies – not quite enough. So, to make things even more diverse, when the gene segments are joined together, additional DNA bases are added or deleted. When this junctional diversity is included, there is no problem creating 100 million B cells, each of which can make a different antibody. The magic of this scheme is that by using modular design and junctional diversity, only a small number of gene segments (about 300) is required to create incredible antibody diversity.

WHAT ANTIBODIES DO

Interestingly, although antibodies are very important in the defense against invaders, they really don't kill anything. Their job is to plant the "kiss of death" on an invader – to tag it for destruction. If you go to a fancy wedding, you'll usually pass through a receiving line before you are allowed to have at the champagne. Of course, one of the functions of this receiving line is to introduce everyone to the bride and groom. But the other function is to be sure no outsiders are admitted to the celebration. As you pass through the line, you will be screened by someone who is familiar with all the invited guests. If she finds that you don't belong there, she will call the bouncer and have you removed. She doesn't do it herself – certainly not. Her role is to identify undesirables, not to show them the door. It's the same with antibodies: They identify invaders, and let other players do the dirty work.

In developed countries, the invaders we encounter most frequently are bacteria and viruses. Antibodies can bind to both types of invaders and tag them for destruction. Immunologists like to say that antibodies can "opsonize" these invaders. This term comes from a German word that means "to prepare for eating." I like to equate opsonize with "decorate," because I picture these bacteria and viruses with antibodies hanging all over them, decorating their surfaces. Anyway, when antibodies opsonize bacteria or viruses, they do so by binding to the invader with their Fab regions, leaving their Fc tails available to bind to Fc receptors on the surface of cells like macrophages. In this way, the antibodies form a bridge between the invader and the phagocyte (e.g., a macrophage), bringing the invader in close, and preparing it for eating (phagocytosis).

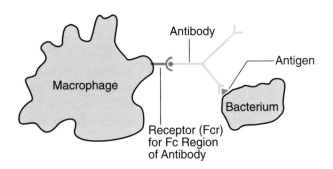

In fact, it's even better than this. When a phagocyte's Fc receptors bind to antibodies that are opsonizing an invader, the appetite of the phagocyte increases, making it even more phagocytic.

During a viral invasion, antibodies can do something else that is very important. Viruses are parasites that enter our cells by binding to certain receptor molecules on the cell's surface. Of course, these receptors are not placed there for the convenience of the virus. They are normal receptors, like the Fc receptor, that have quite legitimate functions, but which the virus has learned to use to its own advantage. Once inside the cell, a virus uses the cellular machinery to make many copies of itself. These newly made viruses then burst out of the cell, sometimes killing it, and go on to infect neighboring cells. Now the neat part. Antibodies can actually bind to a virus while it is still outside of a cell, and can keep the virus either from entering or from replicating once it has entered. Antibodies with these properties are called "neutralizing" antibodies. For example, some neutralizing antibodies can bind to the part of the virus that would plug into the cellular receptor, preventing the virus from "docking" on the surface of the cell. When this happens, the virus is "hung out to dry," opsonized and ready to be eaten by phagocytes!

T CELLS

Although antibodies can tag viruses for phagocytic ingestion, and can help keep viruses from infecting cells, there is a flaw in the antibody defense against viruses: Once a virus gets into a cell, antibodies can't get to it, so the virus is safe to make thousands of copies of itself. Mother Nature recognized this problem, and to deal with it, she invented the famous "killer T cell," another member of the adaptive immune system team.

The importance of T cells is suggested by the fact that in a human, there are about a trillion of them. T cells are very similar to B cells in appearance. In fact, even under a microscope, an immunologist can't tell them apart. Like B cells, T cells are produced in the bone marrow, and they display on their surfaces antibody-like molecules called T cell receptors (TCRs). Like the B cell's receptors (the antibody molecules attached to its surface), TCRs are also made by a mix and match, modular design strategy. As a result, TCRs are about as diverse as BCRs. T cells also obey the principle of clonal selection: When a T cell's receptors bind to their cognate antigen, the T cell proliferates to build up a clone of T cells with the same specificity. This proliferation stage takes about a week to complete, so like the antibody response, the T cell response is slow and specific.

Although they are similar in many ways, there are also important differences between B cells and T cells. Whereas B cells mature in the bone marrow, T cells mature in the thymus (that's why they're called "T" cells). Further, although B cells make antibodies that can recognize any organic molecule, T cells only recognize protein antigens. In addition, the B cell can export (secrete) its receptors in the form of antibodies, but the TCR stays tightly glued to the surface of the T cell. Perhaps most importantly, a B cell can recognize an antigen "by itself," whereas a T cell, like an old English gentleman, will only recognize an antigen if it is "properly presented" by another cell. I'll explain what this means in a bit.

There are actually three kinds of T cells: killer T cells (frequently called cytotoxic lymphocytes – CTLs for short), helper T cells, and regulatory T cells. The killer T cell is a potent weapon that can destroy virus-infected cells. The way it does this is by making contact with its target cell and then triggering it to commit suicide! This "assisted suicide" is a great way to deal with viruses that have infected cells, because when the virus-infected cell dies, the viruses within the cell die with it.

The second type of T cell is the helper T cell (Th cell). As you will see, this cell serves as the quarterback of the immune system team. It directs the action by secreting protein molecules called cytokines that have dramatic effects on other immune system cells. These cytokines have names like interleukin 2 (IL-2) and interferon gamma (IFN-γ), and we will discuss what they do

in later lectures. For now, it is only important to realize that helper T cells are cytokine factories.

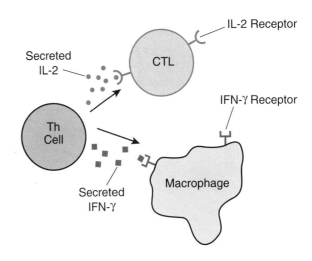

The third type of T cell, the regulatory T cell, is still quite mysterious. It has been very difficult for immunologists to study these cells, in part because unique surface markers have not been identified that would allow regulatory T cells to be easily picked out in a crowd of other T cells. Although it is believed that regulatory T cells may help keep other T cells "under control" (whatever that means), it isn't clear how they do this. Because it is difficult to say at this time how regulatory T cells work, we will focus our attention on killer and helper T cells – cells about which much more is known.

ANTIGEN PRESENTATION

One thing I need to clear up is exactly how antigen is presented to T cells. It turns out that special proteins called major histocompatibility complex proteins (MHC for short) actually do the "presenting," and that T cells use their receptors to "view" this presented antigen. As you may know, "histo" means tissue, and these major histocompatibility proteins, in addition to being presentation molecules, are also involved in the rejection of transplanted organs. In fact, when you hear that someone is waiting for a "matched" kidney, it's the MHC molecules of the donor and the recipient that the transplant surgeon is trying to match.

There are two types of MHC molecules, called class I and class II. Class I MHC molecules are found in varying amounts on the surfaces of most cells in the body, and they function as "billboards" that inform killer T cells about what is going on inside other cells. For example, when a human cell is infected by a virus, fragments of viral proteins (called "peptides") are loaded onto class I MHC molecules, and transported to the surface of the infected cell. By inspecting these protein fragments displayed by class I MHC molecules, killer T cells can use their receptors to look "into" the cell to determine that it has been infected and should be destroyed.

Class II MHC molecules also function as billboards, but this display is intended for the enlightenment of helper T cells. Only certain cells in the body make class II MHC molecules, and these are called "antigen presenting cells" (APCs for short). Macrophages, for example, are excellent antigen presenting cells. During a bacterial infection, a macrophage will "eat" the bacteria, and will load fragments of ingested bacterial proteins onto class II MHC molecules for display on the surface of the macrophage. By using their T cell receptors, helper T cells then can scan the macrophage's class II MHC billboards for news of the bacterial infection. So class I MHC molecules alert killer T cells when something isn't right inside a cell, and class II MHC molecules displayed on APCs inform helper T cells that problems exist outside of cells.

Although a class I MHC molecule is made up of one long chain (the heavy chain) plus a short chain (β2-microglobulin), and class II has two long chains (α and β), you'll notice that these molecules look rather similar.

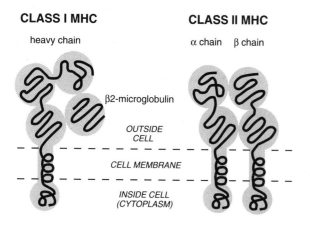

CLASS I MHC

heavy chain

CLASS II MHC

α chain β chain

β2-microglobulin

OUTSIDE CELL

CELL MEMBRANE

INSIDE CELL (CYTOPLASM)

Now I know it's hard to visualize the real shapes of molecules from drawings like this, so I thought I'd show you a few pictures that may make this more real. Here's what an empty MHC molecule might look like from the viewpoint of the T cell receptor. Right away

you see the groove into which the protein fragment would fit.

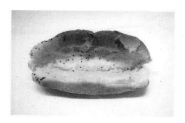

Next, let's look at a fully-loaded, class I molecule:

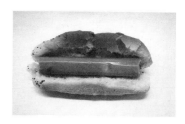

I can tell it's class I because the peptide is contained nicely within the groove. It turns out that the ends of class I molecules are closed, so the protein fragment must be about nine amino acids in length to fit in properly. Class II molecules are slightly different:

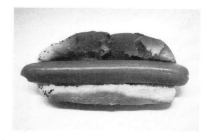

Here you see that the peptide overflows the groove. This works fine for class II, because the ends of the groove are open, so protein fragments as large as about fifteen amino acids fit nicely.

So MHC molecules resemble buns, and the protein fragments resemble wieners. And if you imagine that the cells in our bodies have hot dogs on their surfaces, you won't be far wrong about antigen presentation. That's certainly the way I picture it!

ACTIVATION OF THE ADAPTIVE IMMUNE SYSTEM

Because B and T cells are such potent weapons, Mother Nature put into place the requirement that cells of the adaptive immune system must be activated before they can function. Collectively, B and T cells are called lymphocytes, and how they are activated is one of the key issues in immunology. To introduce this concept, I want to sketch how helper T cells are activated.

The first step in the activation of a helper T cell is recognition of its cognate antigen (e.g., a fragment of a bacterial protein) displayed by class II MHC molecules on the surface of an antigen presenting cell. But the recognition of presented antigen isn't enough – a second signal or "key" is also required for activation. This second signal is non-specific (it's the same for any antigen), and it involves a protein (B7 in this drawing) on the surface of an antigen presenting cell that plugs into its receptor on the surface of the helper T cell (CD28 in this drawing).

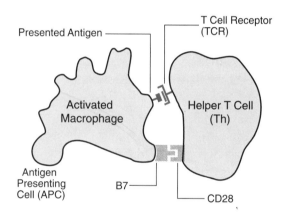

You see an example of this kind of two-key system when you visit your safe deposit box. You bring with you a key that is specific for your box – it won't fit any other. The bank teller provides a second, master key that will fit all the boxes. Only when both keys are inserted into the locks on your box can it be opened. Your specific key alone won't do it, and the teller's non-specific key alone won't either. You need both. Now, why do you suppose helper T cells and other cells of the adaptive immune system require two keys for activation? For safety, of course – just like your bank box. These cells are powerful weapons that must only be activated at the appropriate time.

Once a helper T cell has been activated by this two-key system, it proliferates to build up a clone composed of many helper T cells that recognize the same antigen. These helper cells then mature into cells that can produce the cytokines needed to direct the immune system.

THE SECONDARY LYMPHOID ORGANS

If you've been thinking about how the adaptive immune system might get turned on during an attack, you've probably begun to wonder whether this could ever happen. After all, there are probably only about 10,000 T cells that will have TCRs specific for a given invader, and for these T cells to be activated, they must come in contact with an antigen presenting cell that has also "seen" the invader. Given that these T cells and APCs are spread all over the body, it would seem very unlikely that this would happen before an invasion got completely out of hand. Fortunately, to make this system work with reasonable probability, Mother Nature invented the "secondary lymphoid organs," the most well known of which is the lymph node. You may not be familiar with the lymphatic system, so I'd better say a few words about it.

In your home, you have two plumbing systems. The first supplies the water that comes out of your faucets. This is a pressurized system with the pressure being provided by a pump. In addition, you also have another plumbing system that includes the drains in your sinks, showers, and toilets. This second system is not under pressure – the water just flows down the drain and out into the sewer. The two systems are connected in the sense that eventually the waste water is recycled and used again.

The plumbing in a human is very much like this. We have a pressurized system (the cardiovascular system) in which blood is pumped around the body by the heart. Everybody knows about this one. But we also have another plumbing system, the lymphatic system. This system is not under pressure, and it drains the fluid (called lymph) that leaks out of our blood vessels into our tissues. Without this system, our tissues would fill up with fluid and we'd look like the Pillsbury Doughboy. Fortunately, lymph is collected from our tissues into lymphatic vessels, and is transported by these vessels, under the influence of muscular contraction, through a series of one-way valves to the upper torso, where it is recycled back into the blood. From this diagram, you can see that as the lymph winds its way back to empty into the blood, it passes through a series of way stations, the lymph nodes:

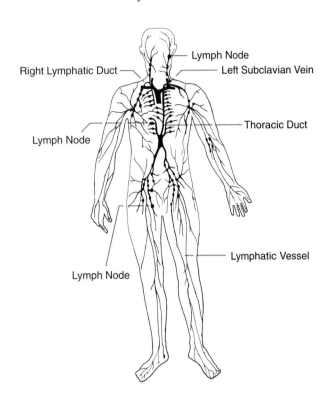

There are thousands of lymph nodes that range in size from very small to almost as big as a brussels sprout. Invaders like bacteria and viruses are carried by the lymph to nearby nodes, and antigen presenting cells that have picked up foreign antigens in the tissues travel to lymph nodes to present their cargo. Meanwhile, T cells and B cells circulate from node to node, looking for the antigens for which they are "fated." So lymph nodes really function as "dating bars" – places where T cells, B cells, APCs, and antigen all gather for the purposes of communication and activation. By bringing these cells and antigens together in the small volume of a lymph node, Mother Nature increases the probability that they will interact to efficiently activate the adaptive immune system.

IMMUNOLOGICAL MEMORY

After B and T cells have been activated, have proliferated to build up clones of cells with identical antigen specificities, and have vanquished the enemy, most of them die off. This is a good idea, because we wouldn't want our immune systems to fill up with old B and T cells. On the other hand, it would be nice if some of these experienced B and T cells would stick around, just in case we are exposed to the same invaders again. That way, the adaptive immune system wouldn't have to start from scratch. And that's just the way it works. These "leftover" B and T cells are called memory cells, and in addition to being more numerous than the original, inexperienced B and T cells, memory cells are also easier to activate. As a result of this immunological memory, the adaptive system usually can spring into action so quickly during a second attack that you never even experience any symptoms.

TOLERANCE TO SELF

As I mentioned earlier, B cell receptors and T cell receptors are so diverse that they should be able to recognize any potential invader. This raises a problem, however, because if the receptors are this diverse, many of them are certain to recognize our own "self" molecules (e.g., the molecules that make up our cells, or proteins like insulin that circulate in our blood). If this were to happen, our adaptive immune system might attack our own bodies, and we could die from autoimmune disease. Fortunately, Mother Nature has devised ways to educate B cells and T cells to discriminate between ourselves and dangerous invaders. Exactly how lymphocytes are taught to be tolerant of self is still being studied, and when this important riddle is finally solved, Nobel Prizes will certainly be awarded. Fortunately, although the mechanisms responsible for self tolerance are still not completely understood, the education which B and T cells receive in self tolerance is sufficiently rigorous that serious attacks on self that result in autoimmune disease are relatively rare.

A COMPARISON OF THE INNATE AND ADAPTIVE IMMUNE SYSTEMS

Now that you have met some of the main players, I want to emphasize the differences between the innate and adaptive immune system "teams." Understanding how they differ is crucial to understanding how the immune system works.

Imagine that you are in the middle of town and someone steals your shoes. You look around for a store where you can buy another pair, and the first store you see is called Charlie's Custom Shoes. This store has shoes of every style, color, and size, and the salesperson is able to fit you in exactly the shoes you need. However, when it comes time to pay, you are told that you will have to wait a week or two to get your shoes – they will have to be custom-made for you, and that will take a while. But you need shoes right now! You are barefoot, and you at least need something to put on your feet until those custom shoes arrive. So they send you across the street to Freddie's Fast Fit – a store that has only a few styles and sizes. Freddie's wouldn't be able to fit Michael Jordan, but this store does stock shoes in the common sizes that fit most people, so you can get a pair right away to tide you over.

This is very similar to the way the innate and adaptive immune systems work. The players of the innate system (like the macrophage) are already in place, and are ready to defend against relatively small quantities of the invaders we are likely to meet on a day-to-day basis. In many instances, the innate system is so effective and so fast that the adaptive immune system never even kicks in. In other cases, the innate system may be overwhelmed, and the adaptive system will be mobilized. This takes a while, because although the B and T cells of the adaptive system can deal with huge quantities of almost any invader, these weapons must be custom-made. Meanwhile, the adaptive immune system must do its best to tide us over by holding the invaders at bay.

THE INNATE SYSTEM RULES!

Until recently, immunologists thought that the only function of the innate system was to provide a rapid defense which would deal with invaders while the adaptive immune system was getting cranked up. However, it is now clear that the innate system does much more than that.

The adaptive immune system's receptors (TCRs and BCRs) are so diverse that they can probably react to any protein molecule in the universe. However, the adaptive system is clueless as to which of these molecules is dangerous and which is not. So how does the adaptive system distinguish friend from foe? The

answer is that it relies on the judgement of the innate system.

In contrast to the receptors of the adaptive immune system, which are totally "unfocused," the receptors of the innate system are precisely tuned to detect the presence of the common pathogens (disease-causing agents) we encounter in daily life – viruses, bacteria, fungi, and parasites. In addition, the innate system has receptors that can detect when pathogens that are "uncommon" (e.g., a new virus) damage human cells. Consequently, it is the innate system that is responsible for sensing danger and for activating the adaptive immune system.

So in a real sense, the innate system gives "permission" to the adaptive system to respond to an invasion. But it's even better than that, because the innate system does more than just "turn the adaptive system on." The innate system actually "integrates" all the information it collects about the invader, and then formulates a plan of action. This "game plan," which is delivered to the adaptive system, tells which weapons to mobilize (e.g., B cells or killer T cells) and exactly where in the body these weapons should be deployed. So if we think of the helper T cell as the quarterback of the adaptive immune system team, we should consider the innate immune system to be the "coach" – for it is the innate system which "scouts" the opponents, designs the game plan, and sends in the plays for the quarterback to call.

EPILOGUE

We have come to the end of our turbo overview of the immune system, and by now you should have a rough idea of how the system works. In the next six lectures, we will focus more sharply on the individual players of the innate and adaptive system teams, paying special attention to how and where these players interact with each other to make the system function efficiently. Then, in the final lectures, we will examine the roles that the immune system plays in disease.

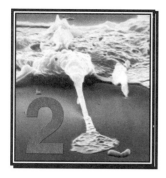

THE INNATE IMMUNE SYSTEM

Until recently, most immunologists didn't pay much attention to the innate system, perhaps because the adaptive system seemed more exciting. However, studies of the adaptive immune system have led to a new appreciation of the role that the innate system plays, not only as a lightning-fast, second line of defense (if we count physical barriers as our first defense), but also as an activator and a controller of the adaptive immune system.

It's easy to understand the importance of the innate system's quick response to common invaders if you think about what could happen in an uncontrolled bacterial infection. Imagine that the splinter from your hot tub deck introduced just one bacterium into your tissues. As you know, bacteria multiply very quickly. In fact, a single bacterium doubling in number every thirty minutes could give rise to roughly 100 trillion bacteria in one day. If you've ever worked with bacterial cultures, you know that a one liter culture containing one trillion bacteria is so dense you can't see through it. So, a single bacterium proliferating for one day could yield a dense culture of about 100 liters. Now remember that your total blood volume is only about five liters, and you can appreciate what an unchecked bacterial infection could do to a human! Without the quick-acting innate immune system to defend us, we would clearly be in big trouble.

The innate immune system includes the complement proteins, professional phagocytes, and natural killer cells. We'll begin our discussion with one of my favorites:

THE COMPLEMENT SYSTEM

The complement system is composed of about twenty different proteins that work together to destroy invaders and to signal other immune system players that the attack is on. The complement system is very old.

Even sea urchins, which evolved about 700 million years ago, have a complement system. In humans, complement proteins start to be made during the first trimester of fetal development, so it's clear that Mother Nature wants this important system to be ready to go, well before a child is born. Indeed, those rare humans born with a defect in one of the complement proteins do not live long before succumbing to infection.

When I first read about the complement system, I thought it was way too complicated to even bother understanding. But as I studied it further, I began to realize that it is really quite simple and beautiful. As with just about everything else in the immune system, the complement system must be activated before it can function, and there are three ways this can happen. The first, the so-called "classical" pathway, depends on antibodies for activation, so we'll leave this for a later lecture. The way the complement system functions is independent of how it is activated, so you won't miss much by waiting until later to hear about the antibody-dependent pathway of activation.

The second way the complement system can be activated is called the "alternative" pathway, although in evolutionary terms, the alternative pathway certainly evolved before the classical pathway. Immunologists call the antibody-dependent system "classical" simply because it was discovered first. Until recently, immunologists thought that these were the only two ways the complement system could be activated. However, a third mode of activation has now been discovered: the "lectin" activation pathway.

THE ALTERNATIVE PATHWAY

The proteins that make up the complement system are produced mainly by the liver, and are present at high concentrations in blood and tissues. The most abundant complement protein is called C3, and in the human body, C3 molecules are continuously being broken into two smaller proteins. One of the protein fragments created by this "spontaneous" cleavage, C3b, is very reactive, and can bind to either of two common chemical groups (amino or hydroxyl groups). Because many of the proteins and carbohydrates that make up the surfaces of invaders (e.g., bacterial cells) have amino or hydroxyl groups, there are lots of targets for these little C3b "grenades."

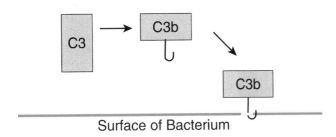

Surface of Bacterium

If C3b doesn't react with one of these chemical groups within about sixty microseconds, it is neutralized by binding to a water molecule, and the game is over. So the spontaneously-clipped C3 molecule has to be right up close to the surface of a cell in order for the complement cascade to continue. Once C3b is stabilized by binding to the cell surface, another complement protein, B, binds to C3b, and complement protein D comes along and clips off part of B to yield C3bBb.

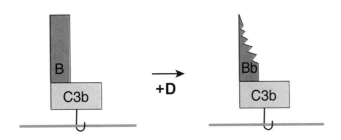

Once a bacterium has this C3bBb molecule glued to its surface, the fun really begins, because C3bBb acts like a "chain saw" that can cut other C3 proteins and convert them to C3b. Consequently, C3 molecules that are in the neighborhood don't have to wait for spontaneous clipping events to convert them to C3b – the C3bBb molecule (called a "convertase") can do the job very efficiently. And once another C3 molecule has been clipped, it too can bind to an amino or hydroxyl group on the surface of the bacterium.

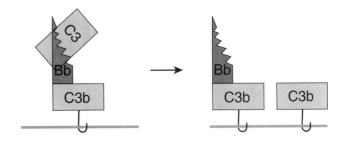

This process can continue, and pretty soon there will be lots of C3b molecules attached to the surface of the target bacterium – and each of them can form a C3bBb convertase that can then cut even more C3 molecules. As you can see, all this attaching and cutting sets up a positive feedback loop, and now the whole thing just snowballs:

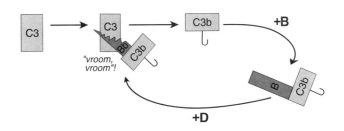

Once C3b is bound to the surface of a bacterium, the complement cascade can proceed further. The C3bBb chain saw can cut off part of another complement protein, C5, and the clipped product, C5b, can combine with other complement proteins (C6, C7, C8, and C9) to make a "membrane attack complex" (MAC for short). To form this structure, C5b, C6, C7, and C8 form a "stalk" that anchors the complex in the bacterial cell wall. Then C9 proteins are added to make a channel that opens up a hole in the surface of the bacterium. And once a bacterium has holes in its surface, it's toast!

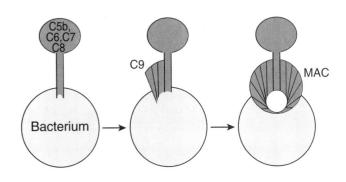

Now, you may be wondering: With these grenades going off all over the place, why doesn't the complement system form MACs on the surface of our own cells? The answer is that human cells are equipped with many safeguards that keep this from happening. In fact, Mother Nature was so worried about the complement system reacting inappropriately that she devoted about as many proteins to controlling the complement system as there are proteins in the system itself. For instance, there is a protein on the surface of human cells called decay accelerating factor (DAF), which accelerates the breakdown of the convertase C3bBb by other proteins in the blood. This can keep the positive feedback loop from getting started. The complement fragment C3b can be clipped to an inactive form by proteins in the blood, and this clipping is accelerated by an enzyme that is present on the surface of human cells. And another cell-surface protein, CD59 (also called protectin), can kick almost-finished MACs off before they can make a hole.

There's an interesting story that illustrates why these safeguards are so important. As you know, transplant surgeons don't have enough human organs to satisfy the demand for transplantation, so they are considering using organs from animals. One of the hot candidates for an organ donor is the pig, because pigs are cheap to raise, and their organs are about the same size as those of humans. As a warm-up for human transplantation, surgeons decided to transplant a pig organ into a baboon. The result was not a big success. Almost immediately, the baboon's immune system began to attack the organ, and within minutes the transplanted organ was a bloody pulp. The culprit? The complement system. It turns out that the pig versions of DAF and CD59 don't work to control primate complement, so the unprotected pig organ was vulnerable to attack by the baboon's complement system.

This story highlights two important features of the complement system. First, the complement system works very fast. These complement proteins are present at high concentrations in blood and in tissues, and they are ready to go against any invader that has a surface with a spare hydroxyl or amino group. A second characteristic of this system is that if a cell surface is not protected, it will be attacked by complement. In fact, the picture you should have is that the complement system is continually dropping these little grenades, and any unprotected surface will be a target. In this system, the default option is death!

THE LECTIN ACTIVATION PATHWAY

In addition to the classical (antibody-dependent) and alternative (antibody-independent) pathways of complement activation, there is a third, recently discovered pathway that may be the most important activation pathway of all. The central player in this pathway is a protein that is produced mainly in the liver, and which is present in moderate concentrations in the blood and tissues. This protein is called mannose-binding lectin (MBL for short). A lectin is a protein that is able to bind to a carbohydrate molecule, and mannose is a carbohydrate molecule found on the surfaces of many common pathogens. For example, mannose-binding lectin has been shown to bind to yeasts such as *Candida albicans*, to viruses such as HIV and influenza A, to many bacteria including *Salmonella* and *Streptococci*, and to parasites like *Leishmania*. In contrast, mannose-binding lectin does not bind to the carbohydrates found on healthy human cells and tissues.

The way mannose-binding lectin works to activate the complement system is very simple. In the blood, MBL binds to another protein called MASP. Then, when the mannose-binding lectin grabs its target (mannose on the surface of a bacterium, for example), the MASP protein functions like a convertase to clip C3 complement proteins to make C3b. Because C3 is so abundant in the blood, this happens very efficiently. The C3b fragments can then bind to the surface of the bacterium, and the complement chain reaction we just discussed is off and running.

So, whereas the alternative activation pathway is spontaneous, and can be visualized as "grenades" going off randomly here and there to destroy any unprotected surface, the lectin activation pathway can be thought of as "smart bombs" that are targeted by mannose-binding lectins. This is an example of an important strategy employed by the innate system: The innate system mainly focuses on patterns of carbohydrates and fats that are found on the surfaces of common pathogens.

OTHER FUNCTIONS OF THE COMPLEMENT SYSTEM

In addition to building membrane attack complexes, the complement system has two other functions in innate immunity. When C3b has attached itself to the surface of an invader, it can be clipped by a serum protein to produce a smaller fragment, iC3b. The "i" prefix denotes that this cleaved protein is now inactive for making MACs. However, it is still glued to the invader, and it can prepare the invader for phagocytosis (can opsonize it) in much the same way that invaders can be opsonized by antibodies. On the surface of phagocytes (e.g., macrophages) are complement receptors that can bind to iC3b, and the binding of iC3b-opsonized invaders facilitates phagocytosis. This is an important function, because many invaders have surfaces that are rather "slimy," making them difficult for macrophages to grasp. When these slippery invaders are coated with complement fragments, phagocytes can get a better grip. Thus, a second function of complement is to decorate the surfaces of invaders, thereby acting like a poor man's antibody in opsonization.

The complement system has a third important function: Fragments of complement proteins can serve as chemoattractants – chemicals that recruit other immune system players to the battle site. For example, C3a and C5a are the pieces of C3 and C5 that are clipped off when C3b and C5b are made (let nothing be wasted!). These fragments don't bind to the surface of invaders. Rather they are set free in the tissues where they are active in attracting macrophages and neutrophils, and in activating these cells so they become more potent killers. Interestingly, these fragments, C3a and C5a, are called anaphylatoxins, because they can contribute to anaphylactic shock – something we will talk about in another lecture.

So the complement system is quite multifunctional. It can destroy invaders by building MACs. It can enhance the function of phagocytic cells by tickling their complement receptors. And it can signal other cells that the attack is on. Most importantly, it can do all these things very fast.

PROFESSIONAL PHAGOCYTES

Professional phagocytes are the second arm of the innate system. These cells are called "professionals" because they make their living mainly by eating (phagocytosis). The most important of the professional phagocytes are the macrophages and the neutrophils.

MACROPHAGES

Macrophages can exist in three stages of readiness. In tissues, macrophages are usually found just lounging

and slowly proliferating. In this "resting" state, they function primarily as garbage collectors, taking sips of whatever is around them, and keeping our tissues free of debris. While resting, they express very few class II MHC molecules on their surfaces, so they aren't much good at presenting antigen to helper T cells. This makes sense. Why would they want to present garbage anyway? For the average macrophage, life is pretty boring. They live for months in tissues and just collect garbage.

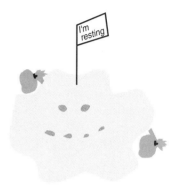

Every once in a while, however, some of these resting macrophages receive signals which alert them that the barrier defense has been penetrated, and that there are intruders in the area. When this happens, they become activated (or "primed," as immunologists usually say). In this state, macrophages take larger gulps and upregulate expression of class II MHC molecules. Now the activated macrophages can function as antigen presenting cells, and when they engulf invaders, they can use their class II MHC molecules to display fragments of the invaders' proteins for helper T cells to see. Although it is likely that a number of different signals can prime a resting macrophage, the best studied is an intercellular communication molecule (a "cytokine") called "interferon gamma" (IFN-γ) that is produced mainly by helper T cells and natural killer (NK) cells.

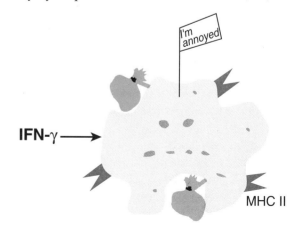

In the primed state, macrophages are good antigen presenters and reasonably good killers. However, they have an even higher state of readiness, "hyperactivation," which they can attain if they receive a direct signal from an invader. For example, such a signal can be conveyed by a molecule called lipopolysaccharide (LPS for short). LPS, a component of the outer cell wall of Gram-negative bacteria like *E. coli.*, can be shed by these bacteria and can bind to receptors on the surface of primed macrophages. Macrophages also have receptors for mannose – the carbohydrate that is an ingredient of the cell walls of many common pathogens and which, as we discussed earlier, is a "danger signal" that can activate the complement system. When receptors on the surface of the macrophage bind to either LPS or mannose, the macrophage knows for sure that there has been an invasion. Faced with this realization, the macrophage stops proliferating, and focuses its attention on killing. In the hyperactive state, macrophages grow larger and increase their rate of phagocytosis. In fact, they become so large and phagocytic that they can ingest invaders that are as big as unicellular parasites. When hyperactivated, macrophages produce and secrete the cytokine tumor necrosis factor (TNF). This cytokine can kill tumor cells and virus-infected cells, and can also help activate immune system cells.

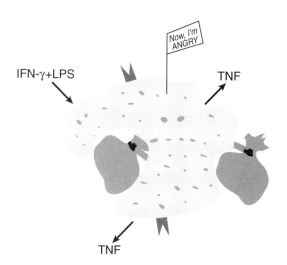

Inside the hyperactivated macrophage, the number of lysosomes increases, so that killing of ingested invaders also becomes more efficient. In addition, hyperactivated macrophages increase production of reactive oxygen molecules like hydrogen peroxide. You know what peroxide can do to hair, so you can imagine what it might do to a bacterium! Finally, when

hyperactivated, a macrophage can dump the contents of its lysosomes onto multicellular parasites, enabling it to destroy invaders that are too large to "eat." Yes, a hyperactivated macrophage is a killing machine!

So a macrophage is a very versatile cell. It can function as a garbage collector, as an antigen presenting cell, or as a vicious killer – depending on its activation level. However, you shouldn't get the impression that macrophages have three "gears." Nothing in immunology has gears, and the activation state of a macrophage is a continuum that really depends on both the type and the strength of the activation signals it receives.

NEUTROPHILS

Although the macrophage is unmatched in versatility, the most important of the professional phagocytes is probably the neutrophil. Neutrophils make up about 70% of the white blood cells in circulation, and about 100 billion of these cells are produced each day in our bone marrow. Clearly they must be important or we wouldn't have so many of them. Neutrophils live a very short time. In fact, they come out of the bone marrow programmed to die in an average of about five days. Interestingly, they die by committing suicide, a process known as "apoptosis." In contrast to macrophages, neutrophils are not antigen presenting cells – they are professional killers. As neutrophils exit the blood, they become activated. In this state, they are very similar to hyperactivated macrophages in that they are incredibly phagocytic, and once their prey has been taken inside, a whole battery of powerful chemicals awaits the unlucky "guest."

My friend Dan Tenen studies neutrophils. His wife, Linda Clayton, who experiments with T cells, likes to kid him by asking, "Why do you bother studying neutrophils? All they do is dive into pus and die!" She's right, of course – pus is mainly dead neutrophils. However, Dan reminds her that humans can live for long periods without those fancy T cells, but without neutrophils, they will succumb to infection and die within a matter of days.

Now, why do you think Mother Nature set things up so that macrophages are very long lived, yet neutrophils live only a few days? Doesn't that seem wasteful? Why not let these neutrophils enjoy a long life, just like the macrophages? That's right! It would be too dangerous. Neutrophils come out of the blood vessels ready to kill, and in the course of this killing, there is always damage to normal tissues. So to limit the damage, neutrophils are programmed to be short lived. If the battle requires additional neutrophils, more can be recruited from the blood – there are plenty of them there. In contrast, you want macrophages to live a long time, because they act as sentinels that watch for invaders and signal the attack.

You may be wondering: If neutrophils are all that dangerous, how do they know when to leave the blood and where to go? It certainly wouldn't do to have neutrophils leave the blood and become activated just any old place. No indeed, and the way this works is really clever. Inside blood vessels, neutrophils exist in an inactive state, and they are swept along by the blood at a high rate of speed: about 1,000 microns per second. If you're the size of a neutrophil, that's really fast.

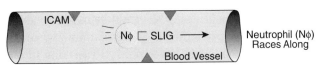

NORMAL TISSUE

In this sketch, you will notice there is a protein, ICAM (short for intercellular adhesion molecule), that is expressed on the surface of the endothelial cells that line blood vessels. There is also another adhesion molecule called selectin ligand (SLIG) that is expressed on the surface of neutrophils. As you can see, however, these two adhesion molecules are not "partners," so they don't bind to each other, and the neutrophil is free to zip along with the flowing blood.

Now imagine that you get a splinter in your big toe, and that the bacteria on the splinter activate macrophages which are standing guard in the tissues of your foot. These activated macrophages give off "alarm" cytokines, interleukin 1 (IL-1) and TNF, which signal that an invasion has begun. When endothelial cells that line nearby blood vessels receive these alarm signals, they begin to express a new protein on their surfaces called selectin (SEL). It normally takes about six hours for this protein to be made and transported to the surface of endothelial cells. Selectin is the adhesion partner for selectin ligand, so when selectin is expressed on the endothelial cell surface, it functions like Velcro to grab neutrophils as they fly by. However, this interaction between selectin and its ligand is only strong enough to cause neutrophils to slow down and roll along the inner surface of the blood vessel.

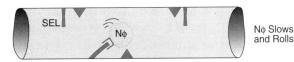

**INFLAMED TISSUE
IL-1 AND TNF**

As the neutrophil rolls, it "sniffs." What it's sniffing for is a signal that there is a battle (an inflammatory reaction) going on in the tissues. The complement fragment, C5a, and the bacterial wall component, LPS, are two of the inflammatory signals that the neutrophil recognizes. When it receives such signals, the neutrophil rushes a new protein called integrin (INT) to its surface. This quick reaction is important, because the neutrophil hasn't stopped – it's still rolling along. If it rolls too far, it will leave the region where selectin is expressed, and the neutrophil will start to zoom along again at "blood speed." To make rapid surface expression of integrin possible, a lot of this protein is made in advance by the neutrophil, and is stored inside the cell until needed.

When integrin appears on the neutrophil's surface, it interacts with its binding partner, ICAM, which is expressed on the surface of endothelial cells. This interaction is very strong, and it causes the neutrophil to stop rolling.

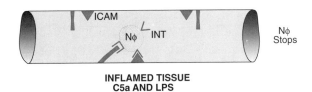

**INFLAMED TISSUE
C5a AND LPS**

Once the neutrophil has stopped, it can be influenced by molecules called chemoattractants to pry apart the endothelial cells that line the blood vessels, exit into the tissues, and migrate to the site of inflammation. These chemoattractants include our old friend from the complement system, C5a, as well as fragments of bacterial proteins called f-met peptides.

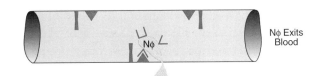

**FOLLOWS "SCENT" OF
f-met AND C5a**

All bacterial proteins begin with a special initiator amino acid called formyl methionine (f-met), which less than 0.01% of human proteins contain, so f-met peptides are relatively unique to bacteria. As they ingest bacteria, macrophages burp up f-met peptides, and neutrophils that have exited the blood can follow the trail of these f-met peptides to find the battle. In addition, cytokines such as TNF activate neutrophils as they travel through the tissues, so they arrive at the battle scene ready to kill.

This system – which involves selectin-selectin ligand binding to make the neutrophil roll, integrin-ICAM interactions to stop the neutrophil, and chemo-attractants and their receptors on the neutrophil to facilitate exit from the blood – may seem a little over-complicated. Wouldn't it be simpler just to have one pair of adhesion molecules (say, selectin and its ligand) do all three things? Yes, it would be simpler, but it would also be very dangerous. In a human there are about 100 billion endothelial cells. Suppose one of them gets a little crazy, and begins to express a lot of selectin on its surface. If selectin binding were the only requirement, neutrophils could empty out of the blood into normal tissues where they could do terrible damage. Having three types of molecules that must be expressed before neutrophils exit the blood helps make the system fail safe.

You remember I mentioned that to completely upregulate expression of that first cellular adhesion molecule, selectin, takes about six hours. Doesn't this seem a bit too leisurely? Wouldn't it be better to begin recruiting neutrophils from the blood just as soon as a macrophage senses danger? Not really. Before you start to recruit reinforcements, you want to be sure that the attack is serious. If a macrophage encounters only a few invaders, it can usually handle the situation without help in a short time. In contrast, a major invasion involving many macrophages can go on for days. The sustained expression of alarm cytokines from many macrophages engaged in battle is required to upregulate selectin expression, and this insures that more troops will be summoned only when they are really needed.

The second feature of this system that I'd like you to notice is that although neutrophils represent about 70% of the white cells in the blood, there are very few neutrophils outside the blood vessels in normal tissues (i.e., tissues that are not infected). Neutrophils are "on call." And who does the calling? The sentinel cell, the macrophage. So here we have this great defense strategy in which garbage collectors alert the "hired guns"

when their help is needed. It is this cooperation between macrophages and neutrophils that makes the whole thing work.

Neutrophils are not the only blood cells that need to exit the blood and enter tissues. For example, eosinophils and mast cells, which are involved in protection against parasites, must exit the blood at sites of parasitic infection. Monocytes, which will eventually become tissue macrophages, also need to leave the blood stream at appropriate places. In addition, T cells and B cells must exit the blood and enter lymph nodes where they can be activated. And once they are activated, T cells and B cells must then be dispatched to sites of infection. This whole business is like a mail system in which there are trillions of packages (immune system cells) that must be delivered to the correct destinations.

This delivery problem is solved in an elegant way by using the same basic strategy that works so well for neutrophils. The key feature of the immune system's "postal service" is that the Velcro-like molecules which cause the cells to roll and stop are different from cell type to cell type and destination to destination. As a result, these cellular adhesion molecules actually serve as "zip codes" to insure that cells are delivered to the appropriate locations. You see, the selectins and their ligands are really families of molecules, and only certain members of the selectin family will pair up with certain members of the selectin ligand family. The same is true of the integrins and their ligands. Because of this two-digit zip code (type of selectin, type of integrin), there are enough "addresses" available to send the many different immune system cells to all the right places. By equipping immune system cells with different adhesion molecules, and by equipping their intended destinations with the corresponding adhesion partners, Mother Nature makes sure that the different types of immune system cells will roll, stop, and exit the blood exactly where they are needed.

NATURAL KILLER CELLS

In addition to the complement system and the professional phagocytes, there is a third important player on the innate immune system team – the natural killer (NK) cell. This has been a difficult cell for immunologists to study, because there are different kinds of NK cells with somewhat different properties. These cells were originally called large granular lymphocytes, because, like the professional phagocytes, they are full of granules that contain chemicals and enzymes. Natural killer cells are descended from stem cells, just like the rest of the blood cells, and are in the same family as the lymphocytes (T and B cells).

Like neutrophils, NK cells use the "roll, stop, exit" strategy to leave the blood and enter tissues at sites of infection. Once in the tissues, NK cells are quite versatile. They can kill tumor cells, virus-infected cells, bacteria, parasites, and fungi. Interestingly, NK cells kill infected cells by forcing them to commit suicide. Sometimes, NK cells employ an "injection system" that uses perforin proteins to deliver "suicide" enzymes (e.g., granzyme B) into the target cell. In other cases, a protein called "Fas ligand" on the NK cell surface interacts with a protein called "Fas" on the surface of the target, signaling the target cell to commit suicide.

One of the mysteries about NK cells is how they identify which cells to kill. Their method of target recognition is quite different from that of killer T cells, which use their T cell receptors to recognize small pieces of invaders. NK cells have no T cell receptors, so they must be looking at something besides peptides displayed by MHC proteins. The latest thinking is that target selection by NK cells involves two signals: a "kill" signal and a "don't kill" signal.

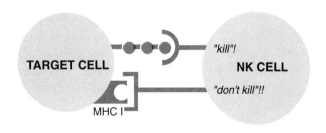

The "don't kill" signal is conveyed by molecules expressed on the surface of the potential target cell. The best studied of these "inhibitory" molecules are our old friends, the class I MHC molecules. Cells that express class I MHC molecules usually can't be killed by NK cells. The "kill" signal is thought to involve interactions between proteins on the surface of the NK cell and special carbohydrates or proteins on the surface of the target cell. Presumably, these unusual surface molecules act as flags that indicate the cell has been infected with a virus or has become a tumor cell, but this part is still poorly understood. The best current synthesis of this two-signal system is that the balance between the "kill" and the "don't kill" signals determines whether NK cells will destroy a target cell.

Now, why do you think it would be a good idea to have NK cells kill targets that do not express class I MHC molecules? You remember that by examining peptides displayed by class I MHC proteins, killer T cells are able to "look inside" cells to see if anything is wrong. But what if some clever virus were to turn off expression of MHC molecules in the cells it infects. Wouldn't those virus-infected cells then be "invisible" to killer T cells? Indeed they would be. So, in those cases, wouldn't it be great to have another weapon that could kill virus-infected cells that don't display MHC molecules on their surfaces? Absolutely. And that's just what NK cells do: They kill cells that lack MHC molecules.

NK cells have a couple of other interesting features. First, in contrast to T cells, which need to be educated not to attack self, NK cells are genius cells that don't need this education. Somehow an NK cell knows an invader when it sees one. It is also notable that NK cells are rather like killer T cells and helper T cells all rolled into one. NK cells can destroy infected cells, just as CTLs can. In addition, like Th cells, NK cells can function as cytokine factories. Indeed, NK cells are one of the major suppliers of IFN-γ.

NK cells also resemble macrophages in some ways. Like macrophages, NK cells contain granules that enclose destructive enzymes and chemicals. In addition, NK cells can exist in several stages of readiness. Resting NK cells produce some IFN-γ and can kill, but they produce more IFN-γ and kill more efficiently if they have been activated. And what activates these killers? Several signals have been identified that can activate natural killer cells, and each of these signals is generated only when the body is under attack. For example, NK cells can be activated when their surface receptors detect the bacterial cell wall component, LPS. NK cells can also be activated by warning proteins called "interferon alpha" and "interferon beta," which are given off by cells when they are being attacked by certain viruses.

THE INNATE IMMUNE SYSTEM – A COOPERATIVE EFFORT

To make the innate system work efficiently, there must be cooperation between players on the innate system team. For example, during a bacterial infection, molecules like LPS bind to receptors on the NK cell surface, signaling that an attack is on. NK cells then respond by producing significant amounts of IFN-γ.

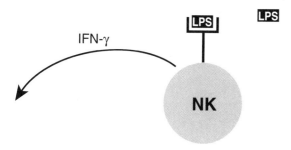

The IFN-γ produced by NK cells can prime macrophages, which can then be hyperactivated when their receptors also bind to LPS.

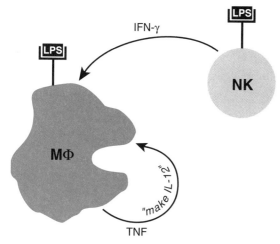

When a macrophage is hyperactivated, it produces lots of TNF. A macrophage also has receptors on its surface to which this cytokine can bind, and when TNF binds to these receptors, the macrophage begins to secrete IL-12. Together, TNF and IL-12 influence NK cells to increase the amount of IFN-γ they produce. And when there is more IFN-γ around, more macrophages can be primed.

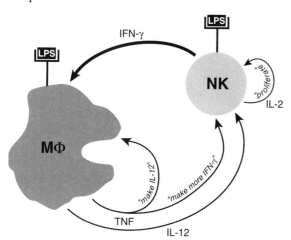

There is something else neat going on here. IL-2 is a growth factor that is produced by NK cells. Normally, however, NK cells don't express the receptor for IL-2, so they don't proliferate in response to this cytokine, even though they are making it. Fortunately, macrophages can fix this problem, because TNF from the macrophage upregulates expression of IL-2 receptors on the surface of NK cells. Consequently, NK cells can now react to the IL-2 they make and begin to proliferate. As a result of this proliferation, there will soon be many more NK cells to defend against an invasion – and to help activate macrophages.

Professional phagocytes and the complement system also work together. As we discussed, complement protein fragments such as C3b can tag invaders for phagocyte ingestion. But complement opsonization can also play a role in activating macrophages, because when C3b fragments that decorate an invader bind to receptors on the surface of a macrophage, this provides an activation signal for the macrophage similar to that supplied by LPS. This is a good idea, because there are invaders that can be opsonized by complement, but which do not make LPS.

Cooperation between the complement system and the phagocytes is not a one-way street. Activated macrophages actually produce several of the most important complement proteins: C3, factor B, and factor D. So in the heat of battle, when complement proteins may be depleted, macrophages can help resupply the complement system. In addition, in an inflammatory reaction, macrophages secrete chemicals that increase the permeability of nearby blood vessels. And when these vessels become leaky, more complement proteins are released into the tissues.

These interactions between phagocytes, NK cells, and the complement proteins are excellent examples of the ways in which innate system players work together. Only by cooperating with each other can the players on the innate system team respond quickly and strongly to an invasion.

HOW THE INNATE SYSTEM DEALS WITH VIRUSES

When viruses enter (infect) human cells, they take over the cells' machinery and use it to produce many more copies of the virus. Eventually, these newly-made viruses burst out of the infected cells, and go on to infect other cells in the neighborhood. We have already discussed some of the weapons the innate system can use to defend against viruses when they are outside of cells. For example, proteins of the complement system can opsonize viruses for phagocytosis by macrophages and neutrophils, and complement proteins can poke holes in enveloped viruses (e.g., HIV-1) by constructing membrane attack complexes on the virus's surface.

Although the innate system is quite effective against viruses when they are <u>outside</u> of cells, once viruses enter cells, the weapons the innate immune system can bring to bear are rather limited. NK cells and activated macrophages secrete cytokines like IFN-γ and TNF that in some cases can reduce the amount of virus that infected cells produce. Secreted TNF also can kill some virus-infected cells, and cells infected by certain viruses can be killed directly by NK cells or by activated macrophages. However, many viruses are quite well protected from the weapons of the innate system once they enter a cell. This is a major problem, because each virus-infected cell can produce thousands of new viruses.

The bottom line here is that complement proteins,

professional phagocytes, and NK cells can help contain a viral infection, especially in the early stages. However, viruses multiply quickly in virus-infected cells, and viruses are very clever. Many have discovered ways of evading the innate system. In fact, it was probably to deal with these rascally viruses that Mother Nature invented the adaptive immune system – the subject of our next three lectures.

SUMMARY FIGURE

In this figure, I have summarized some of the concepts we discussed in this lecture. For clarity, I have chosen a macrophage as a representative of the professional phagocytes, a bacterium as an example of an invader that exists outside human cells, and a virus as an example of a parasite that must enter a human cell to complete its life cycle. After each of the next three lectures, I will expand this figure to include the players from the adaptive immune system as they take the field.

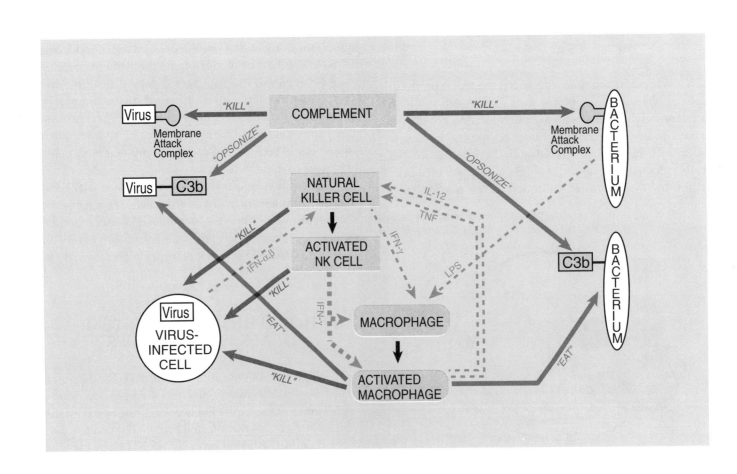

THOUGHT QUESTIONS

1. What is the fundamental difference in the way the complement system is activated by the alternative pathway and by the lectin activation pathway?

2. Why did Mother Nature make macrophages long-lived and neutrophils short-lived?

3. Give examples of the cooperation between players on the innate system team, and tell why this cooperation is important.

4. Describe in words how the innate system deals with a bacterial infection.

5. Describe in words how the innate system deals with a virus attack.

6. What is the main role of the innate system early in an infection?

7. What features of an invader does the innate system recognize?

8. Imagine a splinter has punctured your big toe, and that Gram-negative bacteria have invaded the tissues surrounding the splinter. Sketch the likely sequence of events in which the various players of the innate system team deal with this invasion.

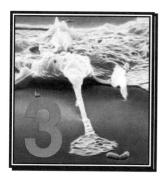

B CELLS AND ANTIBODIES

REVIEW

Let's quickly review the material we covered in the last lecture. We talked about the complement system of proteins, and how complement fragments can function as "poor man's antibodies" to tag invaders for ingestion by professional phagocytes. In addition, complement fragments can act as chemo-attractants to help recruit phagocytic cells to the battle site. Finally, the complement proteins can participate in the construction of membrane attack complexes that can puncture and destroy invading pathogens (e.g., certain bacteria and viruses).

The complement proteins are present in high concentrations in the blood and also in the tissues, so they are always ready to go. In addition, activation by the "alternative" (spontaneous) pathway simply requires that the complement protein fragment, C3b, bind to an amino or hydroxyl group on an invader. Because these chemical groups are ubiquitous, the default option in this system is death – any surface that is not protected against binding by complement fragments will be targeted for destruction.

In addition to the alternative activation pathway, which can be visualized as "grenades" going off randomly here and there, we discussed a second pathway for activating the complement system that is more directed: the lectin activation pathway. In this system, a protein called mannose-binding lectin attaches to carbohydrate molecules that make up the cell walls of common pathogens. Then, a protein that is bound to the mannose-binding lectin sets off the complement chain reaction on the surface of the invader. So the mannose-binding lectin can be thought of as a "smart bomb" that directs the complement system to invaders that have distinctive carbohydrate molecules on their surfaces. We also talked about two professional phago-

cytes: macrophages and neutrophils. In tissues, macrophages have a relatively long lifetime. This makes sense because macrophages act as sentinels that patrol the periphery. If they find an invader, they become "activated." In this activated state, they can present antigens to T cells, can send signals that recruit other immune system cells to help in the struggle, and can become vicious killers.

Whereas macrophages are quite versatile, neutrophils mainly do one thing – kill. Neutrophils use cellular adhesion molecules to exit blood vessels at sites of inflammation, and as they exit, they are activated to become killers. Fortunately, these cells only live about five days. This limits the damage they can do to healthy tissues once an invader has been vanquished. On the other hand, if the attack is prolonged, there are plenty more neutrophils that can exit the blood and help out, since neutrophils represent about 70% of the circulating white blood cells.

Another player on the innate system team is the natural killer cell. These cells are a cross between a killer T cell and a helper T cell. Like CTLs, they can kill virus-infected cells, and like helper T cells, they can secrete cytokines that affect the function of both the innate and the adaptive immune systems.

The innate system is programmed to react to "danger signals" that are characteristic of commonly encountered pathogens or pathogen-infected cells. Phagocytes, natural killer cells, and the complement proteins can attack immediately, because these weapons are already in place. As the battle continues, cooperation between players increases to strengthen the defense, and signals given off by the innate system recruit even more defenders from the blood stream. By working together, the players on the innate system team provide a fast and effective response to common invaders.

The innate system also plays a crucial role in alerting the adaptive immune system to danger. In fact, as we discuss the adaptive system, you will want to be on the lookout for interactions between the innate and adaptive systems. I think you'll soon appreciate that, although its rapid response is crucial for our survival, the innate system does much more than just react quickly.

B CELLS

In this lecture, we will focus on one of the most important adaptive system players: the B cell. Like all the other blood cells, B cells are born in the bone marrow, where they are descended from stem cells. About one billion B cells are produced each day during the entire life of a human, so even old guys like me have lots of freshly made B cells. During their early days in the marrow, B cells select gene segments coding for the two proteins that make up their B cell receptors (BCRs), and these receptors then take up their positions on the surface of the cell. The antibody molecule is almost identical to the B cell receptor, except that it lacks the protein sequences at the tip of the heavy chain that anchor the BCR to the outside of the cell. Lacking this anchor, the antibody molecule is exported out of the B cell (is secreted), and is free to travel around the body to do its thing. I want to tell you a little about the process of selecting gene segments to make a B cell receptor, because I think you'll find it interesting – especially if you like to gamble.

THE B CELL RECEPTOR

The BCR is made up of two kinds of proteins, the heavy chain (Hc) and the light chain (Lc), and each of these proteins is encoded by genes that are assembled from gene segments. The gene segments that will be chosen to make up the final Hc gene are located on chromosome 14, and each B cell has two chromosome 14s (one from Mom and one from Dad). This raises a bit of a problem, because, as we discussed earlier, each B cell makes only one kind of antibody. Therefore, because there are two sets of Hc segments, it will be necessary

to "silence" the segments on one chromosome 14 to keep a B cell from making two different Hc proteins. Of course, Mother Nature could have chosen to make one chromosome a "dummy," so that the other would always be the one that was used to make the Hc protein – but she didn't. That would have been too boring. Instead, she came up with a much sweeter scheme, which I picture as a game of cards with the two chromosomes as players. It's a game of "winner takes all," in which each chromosome tries to rearrange its cards (gene segments) until it finds an arrangement that works. The first player to do this wins.

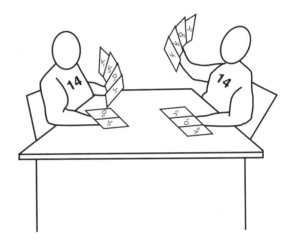

You remember from the first lecture that the finished heavy chain protein is assembled by pasting together four separate gene segments (V, D, J, and C), and that lined up along chromosome 14 are multiple, slightly different copies of each kind of segment.

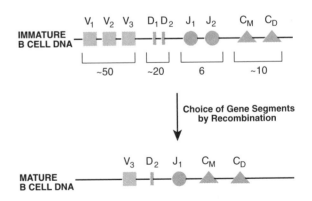

The players in this card game first choose one each of the possible D and J segments, and these are joined together by deleting the DNA sequences in between them. Then one of the many V segments is chosen, and this "card" is joined to the DJ segment, again by deleting the DNA in between. Next to the rearranged J segment is a string of gene segments (C_M, C_D, etc.) that code for various constant regions. By default, the constant regions for IgM and IgD are used to make the BCR, just because they are first in line. Immunologists call these joined-together gene segments a "gene rearrangement," but it is really more about cutting and pasting than rearranging. Anyway, the result is that chosen V, D, and J segments and the constant region segments all end up adjacent to each other on the chromosome.

Next, the rearranged gene segments are tested. What's the test? As you know, protein translation stops when the ribosome encounters one of the three stop codons, so if the gene segments are not joined up just right (in frame), the protein translation machinery will encounter a stop codon and terminate protein assembly somewhere in the middle of the Hc. If this happens, the result is a useless little piece of protein. In fact, you can calculate that each player only has about one chance in nine of assembling a winning combination of gene segments that will produce a full-length, Hc protein. Immunologists call such a combination of gene segments a "productive rearrangement." If one of the chromosomes that is playing this game ends up with a productive rearrangement, the winning Hc protein is made and transported to the cell surface where it signals to the losing chromosome that the game is over. Exactly how the signal is sent and how it stops the rearrangement of gene segments on the other chromosome remain to be discovered.

Since each player only has about a one in nine chance of success, you may be wondering what happens if <u>both</u> chromosomes fail to assemble gene segments that result in a productive rearrangement. Well, the B cell dies. That's right, it commits suicide! It's a high stakes game, because a B cell that cannot express a receptor is totally useless.

If the heavy chain rearrangement is productive, the light chain players step up to the table. The rules of this game are similar to those of the heavy chain game, but there is a second test that must be passed to win: the completed heavy and light chain proteins must fit together properly to make a complete antibody. If the B cell fails to productively rearrange heavy and light chains, or if the Hcs and Lcs don't match up correctly, the B cell commits suicide. So every mature B cell produces one and only one kind of BCR or antibody, made up of one and only one kind of Hc and Lc. Because of the mix and match strategy that is used to make the final

Hc and Lc genes, the receptors on different B cells are so diverse that collectively, they can probably recognize any organic molecule that could exist. When you consider how many molecules that might be, the fact that a simple scheme like this can create such diversity is truly breathtaking.

HOW THE BCR SIGNALS

Immunologists call the antigen that a given B cell's receptors recognize its "cognate" antigen, and the tiny region of the cognate antigen that a BCR actually binds to is called its "epitope." For example, if a B cell's cognate antigen happens to be a protein on the surface of the flu virus, the epitope will be the part of that protein (usually 6 to 12 amino acids) to which the BCR binds. When the BCR recognizes the epitope for which it is matched, it must signal this recognition to the nucleus of the B cell, where genes involved in activating the B cell can be turned on or off. But how does this BCR "antenna" send a signal to the nucleus that it has found its epitope? At first sight it would appear that this could be a bit of a problem, because, as you can see from this figure, the part of the heavy chain that extends through the cell membrane into the interior of the cell is only a few amino acids in length – way too short to do any serious signaling.

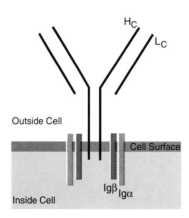

To make it possible for the external part of the BCR to signal what it has seen, B cells are equipped with two accessory proteins, Igα and Igβ, that associate with the heavy chain protein and protrude into the inside of the cell. Thus, the complete B cell receptor really has two parts: the Hc/Lc part outside the cell that recognizes the antigen but can't signal, and the Igα and Igβ proteins that can signal, but which are totally blind to what's going on outside the cell.

To generate a signal, many BCRs must be brought close together on the surface of the B cell. This clustering of BCRs can result when BCRs bind to an epitope that is repeated many times on a single antigen (e.g., a protein in which a sequence of amino acids is repeated many times).

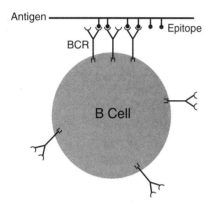

BCRs can also be clustered by binding to epitopes on individual antigens that are close together on the surface of an invader. For example, the surfaces of most bacteria and viruses are made of many copies of a few different proteins. So if a B cell's receptors recognize an epitope on one of these proteins, lots of BCRs can be "focused" on the invader. Finally, B cell receptors can also be brought together by binding to epitopes on antigens that are clumped together (e.g., a clump of proteins). Regardless of how it is accomplished, clustering or "crosslinking" (as immunologists like to say) of B cell receptors is essential for B cell activation. Here's why.

The tails of the Igα and Igβ signaling molecules interact with enzymes inside the cell. When enough of these interactions are concentrated in one region, an enzymatic chain reaction is initiated that sends a message to the nucleus of the cell saying, "BCR engaged." So the trick to sending this message is to get lots of Igα and Igβ molecules together – and that's exactly what clustering of B cell receptors does. The clustering of BCRs brings enough Igα and Igβ molecules together to set off the chain reaction that sends the "BCR engaged" signal. So BCR crosslinking is key.

You remember from last lecture that fragments of complement proteins (e.g., C3b) can bind to (opsonize) invaders. This tag indicates that the invader has been recognized as dangerous by the innate immune system,

and alerts innate system players like macrophages to destroy the opsonized invader. However, it turns out that antigens opsonized by complement fragments can also alert the <u>adaptive</u> immune system. Here's how.

In addition to the B cell receptor and its associated signaling molecules, Igα and Igβ, there is another protein on the surface of a B cell that can play an important role in signaling. This protein is a receptor that can bind to complement fragments which are decorating an invader. Consequently, for an opsonized antigen, there are two receptors on a B cell that can bind to the antigen: the BCR, which recognizes a specific epitope on the antigen, and the complement receptor, which recognizes the "decorations." When this happens, the opsonized antigen acts as a "clamp" that brings the BCR and the complement receptor together on the surface of the B cell.

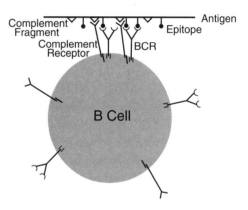

When the BCR and the complement receptor are "crosslinked" in this way by opsonized antigen, the signal that the BCR sends is greatly amplified. What this means in practice is that the number of BCRs that must be clustered to send the "receptor engaged" signal to the nucleus is decreased at least 100-fold. Because the complement receptor can have such a dramatic effect on signaling, it is called a "co-receptor." The function of the co-receptor is especially important during the initial stages of an attack when the amount of antigen available to crosslink B cell receptors is limited. Recognition of opsonized invaders by the B cell co-receptor also serves to make B cells exquisitely sensitive to antigens that the innate system has identified as being dangerous. This is an excellent example of the "instructive" function of the innate system. Indeed, the decision of whether an invader is dangerous or not is generally made by the innate, not the adaptive system.

HOW B CELLS ARE ACTIVATED

To produce antibodies, B cells must first be activated. Most B cells have never encountered their cognate antigen, and these cells are usually called "naive," or "virgin" B cells. An example would be a B cell that can recognize the smallpox virus, but which happens to reside in a human who has never been exposed to smallpox. In contrast, B cells that have already encountered their cognate antigen are termed "experienced." Although both naive and experienced B cells must be activated, the rules for activating these two types of cells are somewhat different, so we will need to focus on them separately. Let's begin with the virgins.

Activation of a naive B cell requires two signals. The first is the clustering of the B cell's receptors and their associated signaling molecules. However, just crosslinking its receptors is not enough to activate a B cell – a second signal is required. Immunologists call this the "co-stimulatory" signal and it is usually provided by a helper T cell (T-cell dependent activation). The best studied co-stimulatory signal involves direct contact between the B cell and the helper T cell. On the surfaces of activated helper T (Th) cells are proteins called CD40L. When CD40L plugs into (ligates) a protein called CD40 on the surface of the B cell, the co-stimulatory signal is sent.

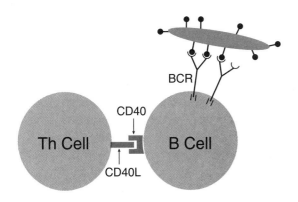

The interaction between these two proteins, CD40 and CD40L, is clearly very important for B cell activation – humans who have a genetic defect in either of these proteins are unable to make a T cell-dependent antibody response.

In response to certain antigens, virgin B cells can also be activated with little or no T cell help. What these antigens have in common is that they have repeated epitopes which can crosslink a ton of B cell receptors. In fact, clustering such a large number of BCRs appears to partially substitute for co-stimulation by CD40L. A good example of such an antigen is a carbohydrate of the type found on the surface of many bacterial cells. A carbohydrate molecule is made up of many repeating units, much like beads on a string. If each "bead" is recognized by the BCR as its epitope, the string of beads can bring together many BCRs and trigger activation. Of course, this type of activation is antigen specific: only those B cells whose receptors recognize the repeated epitope will be activated.

There is another, quite different way that B cells can be activated that is also independent of T cell help. In this case the antigen, usually called a "mitogen," binds to molecules on the B cell surface that are <u>not</u> B cell receptors, clustering these molecules. When this happens, BCRs that are associated with these molecules also are clustered. This "polyclonal" activation is independent of the cognate antigen that is recognized by the BCR – the BCR just comes along for the ride. In this way, many different B cells with many different specificities can be activated by a single mitogen. Indeed, mitogens are favorite tools of immunologists because they can be used to activate a whole load of B cells simultaneously, making it easier to study events that take place during activation.

An excellent example of a mitogen is the highly repetitive structure that makes up the surfaces of certain parasites. B cells have "mitogen receptors" on their surfaces that can recognize these structures. During a parasitic infection, the mitogen receptors on the B cell can be brought close together to focus on the parasite's surface, and when the mitogen receptors are clustered in this way, the BCRs also are clustered. The result is polyclonal activation of B cells that have BCRs on their surfaces which do not recognize the parasite at all.

But why would the immune system want to react to a mitogen (e.g., the surface of a parasite) by activating B cells whose receptors are totally irrelevant? After all, those B cells will be useless in defending against the parasitic attack. The answer is that this is <u>not</u> something the immune system is designed to do! Polyclonal activation is totally unnatural. By activating a bunch of B cells that will produce irrelevant antibodies, the parasite seeks to distract the immune system from focusing on the job at hand – destroying the parasitic invader. So polyclonal activation of B cells is actually an example of the immune system gone wrong – a subject we will discuss at length in another lecture.

I mentioned earlier that the adaptive immune system was designed so that two "keys" are required to activate it. Just as with a safe deposit box, one of these keys is specific. For B cells, this specific key is the crosslinking of B cell receptors. The second key required for activation is nonspecific in that the same key works for all B cells. In the case of T cell-dependent activation, the second key takes the form of the CD40L co-stimulatory molecule that plugs into the CD40 protein on the B cell surface. By making this "two key rule," a fail safe mechanism is established in which the decision to activate is made by a "committee," not by just one cell.

But what about T cell-independent activation of B cells? Doesn't that violate the two-key rule? Sure, a ton of the B cell receptors can be crosslinked by a repeated epitope, but where is the second key? This missing second key has bothered immunologists for some time, because for B cells to be activated simply by recognizing a target with repeated epitopes just seemed too dangerous. So it was a great relief when it was recently discovered that T cell-independent activation really does require two keys.

In careful experiments, immunologists have now shown that when a B cell's receptors are crosslinked, the B cell begins to proliferate. However, after it proliferates, the B cell won't secrete any antibodies – not unless it receives a second signal. And what is this second key? For T cell-independent activation, the second key is a battle cytokine like IFN-γ, which is a clear signal that an attack is on. What this means is that if a B cell recognizes a molecule with repeated epitopes like for example, your own DNA, it may proliferate, but fortunately no anti-DNA antibodies will be produced. The reason is that your immune system is not engaged in a battle with your own DNA, so there will be no battle cytokines available to provide the co-stimulatory signal. On the other hand, if the innate immune system is battling a bacterial infection, and a B cell recognizes a carbohydrate antigen with repeated epitopes on the surface of the bacterial invader, that B cell will produce antibodies, because battle signals (e.g., IFN-γ) generated by the innate system supply the second signal needed for complete B cell activation.

So in response to T-cell independent antigens, B cells can take their cue directly from the innate immune system, and jump right into the battle without having to wait for helper T cells to be activated. The net result is a speedy antibody response to invaders that can activate B cells independent of T cell help.

But there is something else important going on here. Since T cells only recognize protein antigens, if all B cell activation required T cell help, the entire adaptive immune system would be totally focused on proteins. This wouldn't be so great, since many of the most common invaders have carbohydrates or fats on their surfaces that are not found on the surfaces of human cells. Because these carbohydrates and fats are unique to invaders, they make excellent targets for recognition by the immune system. So by allowing some antigens to activate B cells without T cell help, Mother Nature did a wonderful thing: She increased the universe of antigens that the adaptive immune system can react against to include not only proteins, but carbohydrates and fats as well.

As I mentioned, naive and experienced B cells differ in their requirements for activation. In fact, once a B cell has been activated, it remembers that experience, and when it recognizes its cognate antigen again, the requirements for re-activation are less stringent than for the initial activation. The latest thinking is that during re-activation, recognition of cognate antigen is required, but at least in some cases, physical contact between B and Th cells is not necessary.

Now why would it be advantageous to have a system in which it is difficult to activate a B cell for the first time, but relatively easier to re-activate it? Clearly, you want activation of virgin B cells to be tightly controlled, because you only want to activate the adaptive immune system when there is a real threat. So a fail-safe activation requirement for virgin B cells seems reasonable. On the other hand, one of the places you expect to find a lot of experienced B cells is in the collection of memory cells that persists after your first exposure to an invader (e.g., the smallpox virus). These are "legit" B cells that already been through the stringent, two-key selection for primary activation, and as a result are likely to be useful for protection against a second attack. In fact, these are the very B cells that you would like to have activated quickly if you are attacked again. So making it easier for them to be re-activated makes perfect sense.

When B cells have been activated, they express new proteins on their surfaces. One of these is the receptor for IL-2, a growth factor that stimulates B cells to proliferate. What this means is that activation of B cells makes them able to receive cytokine signals that trigger proliferation. This coupling of activation to proliferation forms the basis for clonal selection – only those B cells that have recognized their cognate antigen and have been activated (the selection part) will react to growth factors, proliferate, and form a clone of B cells with identical BCRs. Because the major supplier of growth factors like IL-2 is the helper T cell, T cell help usually is needed for a clone of "selected" B cells to be produced.

Once B cells have been activated and have proliferated to build up their numbers, they are ready for the next stage in their life: maturation. Maturation can be divided roughly into three steps: "class switching," in which the B cell can change the class of antibody it produces; "affinity maturation," in which the rearranged genes for the B cell receptor can undergo mutation and selection that can increase the affinity of the BCR for its cognate antigen; and the career decision in which the B cell decides whether to become an antibody factory (a plasma cell) or a memory B cell. The exact order of these maturation steps varies, and some B cells may skip one or more steps altogether.

CLASS SWITCHING

After B cells are born in the bone marrow, they rearrange the gene segments that encode their heavy and light chain proteins, and they display two classes of antibody molecules on their surfaces: IgM and IgD. These are the BCRs of the young B cell, and usually are called sIgM and sIgD, where the "s" stands for "surface." Interestingly, the same heavy chain mRNA is used to make both sIgM and sIgD, but the mRNA is spliced one way to yield an M-type constant region and another way to produce a D-type constant region. IgD antibodies represent only a tiny fraction of the circulating antibodies in a human, and it is unclear whether these antibodies actually perform any significant function. In contrast, sIgD, found on the surfaces of virgin B cells, is important for B cell activation. Indeed, there are more IgD molecules than IgM molecules on the surface of your average virgin B cell.

When a B cell first leaves the bone marrow, it doesn't secrete antibodies, because it hasn't been activated yet. This virgin B cell must first search for its cognate antigen. If the B cell finds it, and if it receives the co-stimulation it requires (that important second "key"), the B cell will be activated. Once activated, a B cell is ready to produce IgM antibodies – the default antibody class. However, a B cell also has the opportunity to change the class of antibody it makes from IgM to one of the other antibody classes: IgG, IgA, or IgE. You remember that an antibody's class is determined by the constant (Fc) region of its heavy chain – the "tail" of the antibody molecule, if you will. And located just next

to the gene segment that encodes the constant region for IgM are the constant region segments for IgG, IgE, and IgA. So all the B cell has to do to switch its class is to cut off the IgM constant region and paste on one of the other constant regions (deleting the DNA in between). Located between constant region segments on the chromosome are special switching signals that allow this cutting and pasting to take place. For example, here's what happens when a B cell switches from an IgM constant region (C_M in this drawing) to an IgG constant region (C_G).

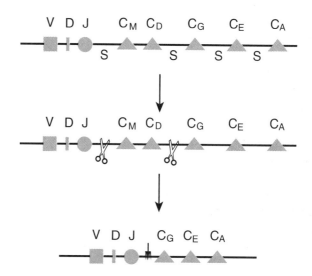

The net result of this switching is that although the part of the antibody that binds to the antigen (the Fab or "hands" region) remains the same, the antibody gets a new tail. This is an important change, because it is the antibody's constant region tail that determines how the antibody will function.

ANTIBODIES AND THEIR FUNCTIONS

Let's take a look at the four main classes of antibodies: IgM, IgG, IgA, and IgE. As you will see, because of the unique structure of its constant (Fc) region, each antibody class is particularly well suited to perform certain duties.

IgM ANTIBODIES

IgM antibodies were the first class of antibodies to evolve, and even "lower" vertebrates (my apologies to the animal rights folks) have adaptive immune systems that produce IgM antibodies. So it makes sense that in humans, when naive B cells are first activated, they mainly make IgM antibodies. You probably remember from the first lecture what an IgG antibody looks like.

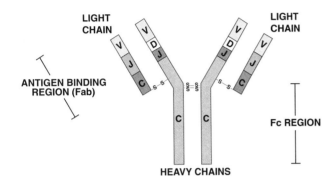

Well, an IgM antibody is like five IgG antibody molecules all stuck together. It's really massive!

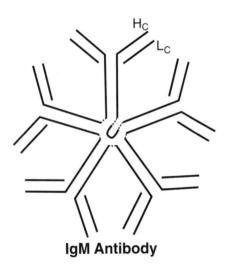

IgM Antibody

Producing this huge IgM antibody early during an infection is quite smart, because IgM antibodies are very good at activating the complement cascade (immunologists call this "fixing complement"). Here's how it works.

In the blood and tissues, some of the complement proteins (about 30 of them!) get together to form a big complex called C1. Despite its size, this complex of proteins cannot activate the complement cascade, because it's bound to an inhibitor molecule. However, if two or more C1 complexes are brought close together, their

inhibitors fall off, and the C1 molecules can then initiate a cascade of chemical reactions that produces a C3 convertase. Now the complement system is in business, because as you remember from the last lecture, the C3 convertase converts C3 to C3b, setting up an amplification loop that produces more and more C3b. So the trick to activating the complement system by this "classical" (antibody-dependent) pathway is to bring two or more molecules of C1 together – and that's just what an IgM antibody can do.

When the antigen binding regions of an IgM antibody bind to an invader, C1 complexes can bind to the Fc regions of the antibody. Because each IgM antibody has five Fc regions close together (this is the important point), two C1 complexes can bind to the Fc regions of the same IgM antibody, bringing the complexes close enough together to set off the complement cascade. So the sequence of events is: The IgM antibody binds to the invader, several C1 molecules bind to the Fc region of the IgM antibody, and these C1 molecules trigger the complement chain reaction on the invader's surface.

This is a nice example of the innate immune system (the complement proteins) cooperating with the adaptive immune system (IgM antibodies) to destroy an invader. In fact, the term "complement" was coined by immunologists when they first discovered that antibodies were much more effective in dealing with invaders if they were "complemented" by other proteins – the complement proteins.

The alternative (spontaneous) complement activation pathway that we talked about in the last lecture is totally non-specific: Any unprotected surface is fair game. In contrast, the classical or antibody-dependent activation pathway is quite specific: Only those antigens to which an antibody binds will be targeted for complement attack. In this system, the antibody identifies the invader, and the complement proteins do the dirty work.

Certain "subclasses" of IgG antibodies can also "fix" complement, because C1 can bind to the Fc region of these antibodies. However, IgG antibodies are real wimps with only one Fc region per molecule. So to bring two C1 complexes close enough together to get things started requires that two molecules of IgG bind very close together on the surface of the invading pathogen – and this is only likely to happen when there is a lot of IgG around. So, early in an infection, when antibodies are just beginning to be made, IgM antibodies have a great advantage over IgG antibodies, because they fix complement so efficiently. In addition, IgM antibodies are very good at "neutralizing" viruses by binding to them and preventing them from infecting cells. Because of these properties, IgM is the perfect "first antibody" to defend against viral or bacterial infections.

IgG ANTIBODIES

IgG antibodies come in a number of different subclasses that have slightly different Fc regions and therefore different functions. For example, one subclass of IgG antibodies, IgG3, fixes complement better than any other IgG subclass. Likewise, the IgG1 subclass is very good at binding to invaders to opsonize them for ingestion by professional phagocytes. This is because macrophages and neutrophils have receptors on their surfaces that can bind to the Fc portion of IgG1 antibodies which have already bound to an invader.

Natural killer cells have receptors on their surface that can bind to the Fc region of IgG3 antibodies. As a result, IgG3 can form a bridge between the NK cell and its target by binding to the target cell (e.g., a virus-infected cell) with its Fab region, and to the NK cell with its Fc region. Not only does this bring the NK cell close to its target cell, but having its Fc receptors bound actually stimulates an NK cell to be a more effective killer. This process is called "antibody-dependent cellular cytotoxicity" (ADCC). In ADCC, the NK cell does the killing, but the antibody identifies the target.

Like IgM antibodies, IgG antibodies are also very good at neutralizing viruses. However, IgG antibodies are unique in that they can pass from the mother's blood into the blood of the fetus by way of the placenta. This provides the fetus with a supply of IgG antibodies to tide it over until it begins to produce its own – several months after birth. This extended protection is possible because IgG antibodies are the longest lived antibody class, with a half life of about three weeks. IgM antibodies have a half life of only about one day.

IgG antibodies are sometimes called "gamma globulins." If there is a possibility that you have been exposed to an infectious agent, say hepatitis A virus, your doctor may recommend that you get a gamma globulin shot. These shots are prepared by pooling together antibodies from a large number of people, at least some of whom have been infected with hepatitis A virus, and are therefore making antibodies against the virus. The hope is that these "borrowed" antibodies will

neutralize most of the virus to which you have been exposed, and that this treatment will at least keep the viral infection under control until your own immune system can be activated.

IgA ANTIBODIES

Here's a question for you: What is the most abundant antibody class in the human body? No, it's not IgG. It's IgA. This is really a trick question, because I told you earlier that IgG was the most abundant antibody class in the blood – which is true. It turns out, however, that we humans synthesize more IgA antibodies than all other antibodies combined. Why so much IgA? Because IgA is the main antibody class that guards the mucosal surfaces of the body, and a human has about 400 square meters of mucosal surfaces to defend. These include the digestive, respiratory, and reproductive tracts. So although there aren't a lot of IgA antibodies circulating in the blood, there are tons of them protecting the mucosal surfaces. Indeed, about 80% of the B cells that are located beneath these surfaces produce IgA antibodies.

One reason IgA antibodies are so good at defending against invaders that would like to penetrate the mucosal barrier is that each IgA molecule is like two IgG molecules held together by a "clip."

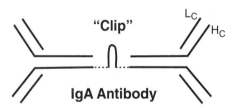

The clipped-together tail structure of IgA antibodies is responsible for several important properties of this antibody class. Because of the clip that holds them together, IgA antibodies can be transported from the blood across the intestinal wall and out into the intestine. Once inside the intestine, IgA antibodies can "coat" invading pathogens and keep them from attaching to the intestinal cells they would like to infect. In addition, whereas each IgG molecule has two antigen binding regions (two "hands"), the "dimeric" IgA molecule has four hands to bind to antigens. Because they are dimeric, IgA antibodies are very good at collecting pathogens together into clumps that are large enough to be swept out of the body with the mucus. In fact, rejected bacteria make up about 30% of the material in normal feces!

Their unique tail structure also makes IgA antibodies resistant to acids and enzymes found in the digestive tract. All together, these qualities make IgA antibodies perfect for guarding mucosal surfaces. Indeed, it is the IgA class of antibodies that is secreted into the milk of nursing mothers. These IgA antibodies coat the baby's intestinal mucosa and provide protection against pathogens that the baby ingests. This makes sense, because many of the microbes that babies encounter are taken in through their mouths – babies like to put their mouths on everything, you know.

Although IgA antibodies are very effective against mucosal invaders, they are totally useless at fixing complement, because C1 won't bind to an IgA antibody's Fc region. Again we see that the constant region of an antibody determines both its class and its function. This lack of complement-fixing activity is actually a good thing. If IgA antibodies could initiate the complement reaction, our mucosal surfaces would be in a constant state of inflammation in response to the pathogenic and non-pathogenic visitors that continuously assault our mucosal surfaces. And having chronically inflamed intestines would not be all that great. So IgA antibodies mainly function as "passive" antibodies that block the attachment of invaders to cells that line our mucosal surfaces, and usher these unwanted guests out of the body.

IgE ANTIBODIES

The IgE antibody class has an interesting history. In the early 1900s, a French physician named Charles Richet was sailing with Prince Albert of Monaco (Grace Kelly's father-in-law). The prince remarked to Richet that it was very strange how some people react violently to the toxin in the sting of the Portuguese Man of War, and he suggested that this phenomenon might be worthy of study.

Richet took his advice, and when he returned to Paris, he decided, as a first experiment to test how much toxin was required to kill a dog. Don't ask me why he decided to use dogs in his experiments. Maybe there were lots of stray dogs around back then, or perhaps he just didn't like mice. Anyway, the experiment was a success and he was able to determine the amount of

toxin that was lethal. However, many of the dogs he used in this first experiment survived because they didn't receive the lethal dose. Not being one who would waste a good dog, Richet decided to inject these "leftovers" with the toxin again to see what would happen. His expectation was that these animals might have become immune to the effects of the toxin, and that the first injection would have provided protection (prophylaxis) against a second injection. You can imagine his surprise then, when all the dogs died – even the ones that received tiny amounts of toxin in the second injection! Since the first injection had the opposite effect of protection, Richet coined the word "anaphylaxis" to describe this phenomenon ("ana" is a prefix meaning "opposite"). Richet continued these studies on anaphylactic shock, and in 1913, he received the Nobel Prize for his work. I guess one lesson here is that if a prince suggests you should study something, you might want to take his advice seriously!

Immunologists now know that anaphylactic shock is caused by mast cells degranulating. Like macrophages, mast cells are white blood cells that are stationed beneath all exposed surfaces (e.g., beneath the skin or the mucosal barrier). As blood cells go, mast cells are very long lived. They can survive for years in our tissues, lying in wait to protect against invaders. Recently, it has been learned that mast cells play a role in the innate defense against bacteria by phagocytosing opsonized bacteria, and by giving off cytokines that recruit neutrophils and other immune system cells to the site of a bacterial infection. However, the most famous function of mast cells is to protect against infection by parasites that have penetrated the barrier defense. Stored safely inside mast cells are lots of granules that contain all kinds of pharmacologically active chemicals, the most famous of which is histamine. When a mast cell encounters a parasite, it dumps the contents of these granules (i.e., it "degranulates") onto the parasite to kill it. However, in addition to killing parasites, mast cell degranulation can also cause an allergic reaction, and in extreme cases, anaphylactic shock. Here's how it works.

An antigen (e.g., the Man of War toxin) that can cause an allergic reaction is called an allergen. On the first exposure to an allergen some people, for reasons that are far from clear, make lots of IgE antibodies directed against the allergen. Mast cells have receptors on their surfaces that can bind to the Fc region of these IgE antibodies, and when this happens, the mast cells are like grenades waiting to explode.

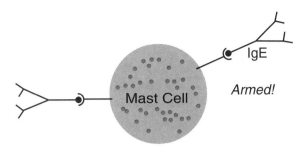

AFTER FIRST EXPOSURE

On a second exposure to the allergen, IgE antibodies that are already bound to the surfaces of mast cells can bind to the allergen. Because allergens are usually small proteins with a repeating sequence, the allergen can crosslink many IgE molecules on the mast cell surface, dragging the Fc receptors together. This clustering of Fc receptors is similar to the crosslinking of B cell receptors in that in both cases, bringing many of these receptors together results in a signal being sent. However, here the signal says "degranulate," and the mast cell dumps its granules into your tissues.

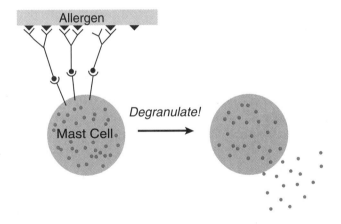

Histamines and other chemicals released from mast cell granules increase capillary permeability, so that fluid escapes from the capillaries into the tissue – that's why you get a runny nose and watery eyes when you have an allergic reaction. This is usually a rather local effect, but if the toxin spreads throughout the body and triggers massive degranulation of mast cells, things can get very serious. In such a case, the release of fluid from the blood into the tissues can reduce the blood volume so much that the heart no longer can pump efficiently, resulting in a heart attack. In addition, histamine

from the granules can cause smooth muscles around the windpipe to contract, making it difficult to breathe. In extreme cases, this contraction can be strong enough to cause suffocation. Around here, we don't worry much about Portuguese Men of War, but we <u>are</u> concerned about bees, because the toxin in a bee sting can cause fatal anaphylactic shock in some people – those individuals who make lots of IgE antibodies in response to bee toxin.

This brings us to an interesting question: Why are B cells allowed to switch the class of antibody they make anyway? Wouldn't it be safer just to stick with good old IgM antibodies?

Let's suppose you have a viral infection of your respiratory tract (e.g., the common cold). Would you want to be stuck making only IgM antibodies? Certainly not. You'd want a lot of IgA antibodies to be secreted into the mucus that lines your respiratory tract to bind up that virus, and remove it from your body. On the other hand, if you have a parasitic infection (say, some sort of worms), you'd want IgE antibodies to be produced, because IgE antibodies can cause cells like mast cells to degranulate, making life miserable for those worms. So the beauty of this system is that the different classes of antibodies are uniquely suited to defend against different invaders.

ANTIBODY CLASS	ANTIBODY PROPERTIES
IgM	Great Complement Fixer Good Opsonizer First Antibody Made
IgA	Resistant to Stomach Acid Protects Mucosal Surfaces Secreted in Milk
IgG	OK Complement Fixer Good Opsonizer Helps NK Cells Kill (ADCC) Can Cross Placenta
IgE	Defends Against Parasites Causes Anaphylactic Shock Causes Allergies

Now suppose Mother Nature could arrange to have your immune system make IgA antibodies when you have a cold, and IgE antibodies when you have a parasitic infection? Wouldn't that be elegant? Well, it turns out that this is exactly what happens! Here's how it works.

Antibody class switching is controlled by the cytokines that B cells encounter when switching takes place: Certain cytokines or combinations of cytokines influence B cells to switch to one class or another. For example, if B cells class switch in an environment that is rich in IL-4 and IL-5, they preferentially switch their class from IgM to IgE – just right for those worms. On the other hand, if there is a lot of IFN-γ around, B cells switch to produce IgG3 antibodies that are very effective against bacteria and viruses. Or, if a cytokine called TGF-β is present during the class switch, B cells preferentially change from IgM to IgA antibody production – perfect for the common cold. So to ensure that the antibody response will be appropriate for a given invader, all Mother Nature has to do is to arrange to have the right cytokines present when B cells switch classes. But how could she accomplish this?

You remember that helper T (Th) cells are "quarterback" cells which direct the immune response. One way they do this is by producing cytokines which influence B cells to make the antibody class that is right to defend against a given invader. To learn how Th cells know which cytokines to make, you'll have to wait for the next two lectures when we discuss antigen presentation and T cell activation. But for now, I'll just give you the bottom line: In response to cytokines made by Th cells, B cells can switch from producing IgM antibodies to producing one of the other antibody classes. This makes it possible for the adaptive immune system to respond with antibodies tailor-made for each kind of invader – be it a bacterium, a flu virus, or a worm. What could be better than that!

SOMATIC HYPERMUTATION

As if class switching weren't great enough, there is yet another amazing thing that can happen to B cells as they mature. Normally, the overall mutation rate of DNA in human cells is extremely low, only about one mutated base per 100 million bases per DNA replication cycle. It has to be this low or we'd all end up looking like Star Wars characters with three eyes and six ears. However, in very restricted regions of the chromosomes of B cells – those regions that contain the V, D, and J gene segments – an extremely high rate of mutation can take place. In fact, mutation rates as high as one mutated base per thousand bases per generation have been measured. We're talking serious mutations here! This high rate of mutation is called "somatic hypermutation," and it occurs after the V, D, and J segments have been selected, and usually after class switching has taken place. So somatic hypermutation is a relatively late event in the maturation of B cells, and B cells that still make IgM antibodies usually have not undergone somatic hypermutation.

What somatic hypermutation does is to change (mutate) the part of the rearranged antibody gene that encodes the antigen binding region of the antibody. Depending on the mutation, there are three possible outcomes: The affinity of the antibody molecule for its cognate antigen may remain unchanged, it may be increased, or it may be decreased. Now comes the neat part. It turns out that for maturing B cells to continue to proliferate, they must be continually re-stimulated by binding to their cognate antigen. Therefore, because those B cells whose BCRs have mutated to higher affinity are stimulated more easily (because their BCRs bind better), they proliferate more frequently than do B cells with lower-affinity receptors. And because B cells with high-affinity receptors proliferate more frequently, the result of somatic hypermutation is that you end up with many more B cells whose BCRs have high affinity for their cognate antigen.

By using somatic hypermutation to make changes in the antigen binding region of the BCR, and by using binding and proliferation to select those mutations that have increased the BCR's ability to bind to antigen, B cell receptors can be "fine tuned." The result is a collection of B cells whose receptors have a higher average affinity for their cognate antigen. This whole process is called affinity maturation.

So B cells can change their constant (Fc) region by class switching and their antigen binding (Fab) region by somatic hypermutation – and these two modifications produce B cells that are better adapted to deal with invaders. Both of these changes are controlled by cytokines that are provided mainly by helper T cells. As a result, B cells that are activated without T cell help (e.g., in response to carbohydrates on the surface of a bacterium) usually don't undergo either class switching or somatic hypermutation.

B CELLS MAKE A CAREER CHOICE

The final step in the maturation of a B cell is the choice of profession. This can't be too tough, because a B cell really has only two fates to choose between: to become a plasma cell or a memory cell. Plasma cells are antibody factories. If a B cell decides to become a plasma cell, it usually travels to the spleen or back to the bone marrow, and begins to produce the secreted form of the BCR – the antibody molecule. Plasma B cells crank out about two thousand of these antibodies each second. The fact that one plasma B cell can make so many antibodies enables the immune system to keep up with invaders like bacteria and viruses, which multiply very quickly. However, as a result of this heroic effort, most plasma B cells live only a few days.

Although the B cell's other possible career choice – to become a memory B cell – may not be quite so dramatic as the decision to become a plasma cell, it is extremely important: It is the memory B cell that remembers your first exposure to a pathogen, and defends you against subsequent exposures. Memory B cells usually have undergone class switching, so they produce the class of antibody that is especially appropriate to defend against the invader they remember. In addition, most memory B cells have experienced somatic hypermutation, so they have high affinity BCRs that can respond to the low levels of antigen that are present at the beginning of an infection. Finally, memory B cells have less stringent activation requirements than do naive B cells. Because of these properties, memory B cells are "ready to go" to defend against a second attack.

It is clear that memory B cells can confer life-long immunity to infection. For example, in 1781 Swedish traders brought the measles virus to the isolated Faeroe islands. In 1846, when another ship carrying sailors infected with measles visited the islands, people who were older than 64 years did not contract the disease – they still had antibodies against the measles virus. How this long-lasting B cell immunity is maintained is currently being debated. Even the longest-lived antibodies (the IgG class) only have a half life of about three weeks, so antibodies must be made continuously to provide long-lasting protection. Some evidence suggests that memory B cells can live a long time. Other experiments indicate that memory B cells are relatively short-lived, but that from time to time they proliferate when they are re-stimulated by antigen. This could be antigen that is left around after the attack, or it might be another antigen that is similar enough to the invader to re-stimulate memory B cells. According to this scenario, it is actually the descendants of the original memory B cells that make the antibodies which confer immunity.

Immunologists also haven't figured out how a B cell "chooses" to become either a memory cell or a plasma cell. However, they do know that the interaction between CD40L on the surface of a helper T cell and CD40 on the B cell surface is important in memory cell generation as well as for class switching and somatic hypermutation. This need for a CD40L-CD40 interaction helps explain why memory B cells usually are not produced when B cells are activated without T cell help, and why T cell-independent activation generally produces IgM antibodies that have not been "refined" by somatic hypermutation.

SUMMARY FIGURE

Our summary figure now includes the innate immune system from the last lecture plus the B cells and antibodies that we discussed here.

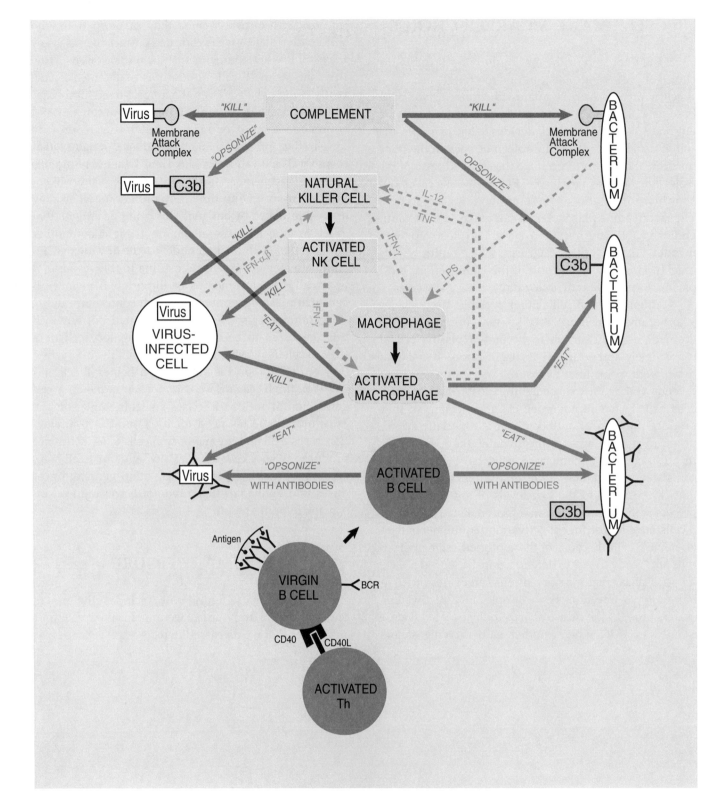

THOUGHT QUESTIONS

1. B cells are produced according to the principle of clonal selection. What does this mean exactly?

2. Describe what happens during T cell–dependent activation of B cells.

3. Describe two "fail safe" systems that are involved in B cell activation.

4. Describe how B cells can be activated without T cell help.

5. Why is T cell–independent activation of B cells important in defending us against certain pathogens?

6. Describe the main attributes of IgM, IgG, and IgA antibodies.

7. Why do class switching and somatic hypermutation produce B cells that are better able to defend against invaders?

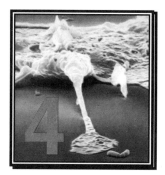

THE MAGIC OF ANTIGEN PRESENTATION

REVIEW

In the last lecture we discussed B cells and antibodies, so let's do a bit of review. A B cell's receptors function as the "eyes" of the cell, and actually have two parts: a recognition part (made up of the heavy and light chain proteins), and a signaling part (made up of two other proteins, Igα and Igβ). The final genes that encode the recognition part are made by mixing and matching gene segments. The result is a collection of B cells with receptors so diverse that they can probably recognize any organic molecule in the universe. For these receptors to signal what they have seen requires that multiple BCRs be clustered (crosslinked). This crosslinking brings the Igα and Igβ signaling molecules that are associated with the heavy chains close together. And when enough Igα and Igβ molecules are clustered in this way, a threshold amount of enzymatic activity is reached, and the "receptor engaged" signal is sent to the nucleus of the B cell.

Activation of a virgin B cell requires two "keys," and crosslinking of the B cell's receptors is the first key. In addition, a second, "co-stimulatory" key also is required. This key usually is provided by a helper T cell, and involves cell-cell contact during which CD40L molecules on the surface of the helper T cell bind to the CD40 proteins on the surface of a B cell. B cells can also be activated without T cell help. The first requirement for this T cell–independent activation is that a ton of the B cell's receptors be crosslinked. This typically happens when the surface of an invader is made up of many copies of the antigen to which a B cell's receptors bind (its "cognate" antigen). Although the crosslinking of many B cell receptors is a requisite for T cell–independent activation of a naive B cell, it is not enough. A second, co-stimulatory signal is also

needed. This co-stimulation is usually supplied by the innate system in the form of "battle cytokines," which bind to other receptors on the surface of the B cell. By demanding that two keys must be supplied before a B cell can be activated, a fail-safe system is established that guards against inappropriate B cell activation.

IgM antibodies are the first antibodies produced by virgin B cells in response to a pathogen that has not been encountered before. However, as a B cell matures, it can choose to produce a different class of antibody: either IgG, IgA, or IgE. This class switching does not change the antigen binding region of the antibody (the Fab or "hands" region). Consequently, the antibody recognizes the same antigen before and after its class has been switched. What does change during class switching is the Fc region of the heavy chain (the "tail" of the antibody, if you will). This is the part of the antibody that determines how the antibody functions, with some of these functions being better suited to certain invaders than to others. Importantly, the choice of antibody class is determined by the cytokines present in the local environment of the B cell when switching takes place. So by arranging to have appropriate cytokines produced at the appropriate places, Mother Nature can insure that the antibodies made will be just right to defend against a particular invader.

The other change that can take place as a B cell matures is somatic hypermutation. In contrast to class switching, in which the antibody gets a new tail, somatic hypermutation alters the antigen binding region of the antibody. Since the probability of a B cell being triggered to proliferate depends on the affinity of its BCR for antigen, B cells in which somatic hypermutation has increased the binding affinity of their

BCRs will proliferate most. Consequently, somatic hypermutation and selection for proliferation results in a collection of B cells whose BCRs bind more tightly to an invader. These cells are especially useful as memory B cells, because their affinity-matured BCRs are so sensitive that they can be reactivated early in a second infection while the number of invaders is still relatively small.

It is important to note that although B cells can be activated with or without T cell help, the outcomes in these two cases are very different. T cell–independent activation mostly results in the production of IgM antibodies. In contrast, T cell–dependent activation usually produces affinity-matured, IgG or IgA antibodies. One reason for this difference is that both class switching and somatic hypermutation are triggered by cytokines, and Th cells are the major sources of these cytokines. Moreover, both processes require ligation of CD40 on B cells by CD40L, a protein found on the surfaces of activated helper T cells.

As B cells mature, they must also decide whether to become short-lived plasma cells that make lots of the secreted form of the BCR that we call antibodies – or to go back to the resting state as longer-lived, memory B cells. Exactly how this decision is made is not clear.

THE MAGIC OF ANTIGEN PRESENTATION

Of all the concepts on which the immune system is based, perhaps the most elegant, and certainly the most unexpected, is antigen presentation: the concept of having one cell present fragments of proteins to another cell. As you will see, antigen presentation is central to the function of the adaptive immune system, with the cells that present antigen to T cells, the "antigen presenting" cells (APCs) playing a pivotal role. Let's begin by discussing the "billboards" on APCs that actually do the presenting: the class I and class II MHC molecules.

CLASS I MHC MOLECULES

The structures of both class I and class II MHC molecules have now been carefully analyzed, so we have a pretty good idea of what both molecules look like. Class I molecules have a binding groove that is closed at both ends, so the small protein fragments (peptides) they present must fit within the confines of the groove (or the "bun," if you will). Indeed, when immunologists pried peptides from the grasp of class I molecules and sequenced them, they found that most of them are 8 to 11 amino acids in length. These peptides are anchored at the ends, and the slight variation in length is accommodated by letting the peptide bulge out a bit in the center.

Every human has three genes for class I MHC proteins (called HLA-A, HLA-B, and HLA-C), located on chromosome six. Because we have two chromosome sixes (one from Mom and one from Dad), we each have a total of six class I MHC genes. Each of the class I HLA proteins pairs with another protein called β2-microglobulin to make up the complete class I MHC molecule.

In the human population, there are many slightly different forms of the genes that encode the three class I HLA proteins. For example, there are at least 125 different variants of the gene for the HLA-A protein. The proteins encoded by these genes all have the same rough shape, but they differ by one or a few amino acids. Immunologists call molecules that have many forms "polymorphic," and the class I HLA proteins certainly fit this description. In contrast, all of us have the same β2-microglobulin protein. It is "monomorphic."

Because they are polymorphic, class I MHC molecules can have different binding motifs, and therefore can present peptides that have different kinds of amino acids at their ends. For example, some class I MHC molecules bind to peptides that have hydrophobic amino acids at one end, whereas other MHC molecules prefer basic amino acids at this anchor position. Since humans have the possibility of expressing up to six different class I molecules, collectively our class I molecules can present a wide variety of peptides. Moreover, although MHC I molecules are picky about binding to certain amino acids at the ends of the peptide, they are rather promiscuous in their selection of amino acids at the center of the protein fragment. As a result, a given class I MHC molecule can bind to and present a large number of different peptides, each of which "fits" the particular amino acids present at the ends of its binding groove.

CLASS II MHC MOLECULES

Like class I molecules, class II MHC molecules (encoded by genes in the HLA-D region of chromosome six) are wildly polymorphic: Within the human population many different versions of class II molecules exist. However, in contrast to class I MHC molecules, the binding groove of class II MHC molecules is open at both ends, so the peptide can hang out of the groove. As you might expect from this feature, peptides that bind to class II molecules are longer than those that occupy the closed groove of class I molecules – in the range of thirteen to twenty-five amino acids. Further, for class II, the critical amino acids that anchor the peptides are spaced along the binding groove instead of being clustered at the ends.

ANTIGEN PRESENTATION BY CLASS I MHC MOLECULES

MHC I molecules are "billboards" that display on the surface of a cell, fragments of proteins manufactured by that cell. Immunologists call these "endogenous" proteins. These include ordinary cellular proteins like enzymes and structural proteins, as well as proteins encoded by viruses and other parasites that have infected the cell. For example, when a virus enters a cell, it uses the cellular biosynthetic machinery to produce proteins encoded by viral genes. A sample of these viral proteins is displayed by class I MHC molecules along with samples of all the normal cellular proteins. So in effect, the MHC I billboards advertise a "sampling" of all the proteins that are being made inside a cell. Almost every cell in the human body expresses class I molecules on its surface, although the number of molecules varies from cell to cell. Killer T cells (also called cytotoxic lymphocytes or CTLs) inspect the protein fragments displayed by class I MHC molecules. Consequently, almost every cell is an "open book" that can be checked by CTLs to determine whether it has been invaded by a virus or other parasite and should be destroyed.

The way endogenous proteins are processed and loaded onto class I MHC molecules is very interesting. Usually, when mRNA is translated into protein in the cytoplasm of a cell, this process goes quite nicely. But sometimes mistakes are made, and the newly minted proteins don't fold up correctly, and therefore are useless. In addition, proteins get damaged as a result of normal wear and tear. So to make sure our cells don't fill up with defective proteins, old or useless proteins are fed into protein-destroying "machines" in the cytoplasm that function rather like wood chippers. These protein chippers are called proteasomes, and they cut

proteins up into small pieces. Most of these peptides are then broken down further into individual amino acids, which are re-used to make new proteins. However, some of the peptides created by the proteasomes are carried by specific transporter proteins (TAP1 and TAP2) across the membrane of the endoplasmic reticulum (ER), a large, sack-like structure inside the cell from which most proteins destined for transport to the cell surface begin their journey.

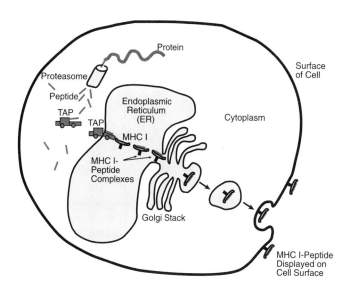

Once inside the ER, some of these peptides are chosen to be loaded into the grooves of class I MHC molecules. I say "chosen," because as we discussed, not all peptides will fit. For starters, a peptide must be the right length – about nine amino acids. In addition, the amino acids at the ends of the peptide must be compatible with the anchor amino acids that line the ends of the groove of the MHC molecule. Obviously, not all of the "chips" prepared by the proteasome will have these characteristics, and those that don't are shipped back out of the ER into the cytoplasm to be broken down further. Once class I MHC molecules are loaded with peptides, they proceed to the surface of the cell for display. So there are three main steps in preparing a class I display: generation of the peptide by the proteasome, transport of the peptide into the ER by the TAP transporter, and binding of the peptide to the groove of the MHC I molecule.

In "ordinary" cells like liver cells and heart cells, the major function of proteasomes is to deal with defective proteins. So as you can imagine, the chippers in these cells are not too particular about how proteins are cut up – they just hack away. As a result, some of the peptides will be appropriate for MHC presentation, but most will not be. In contrast, in cells like macrophages that specialize in presenting antigen, this chipping is not so random. For example, binding of IFN-γ to receptors on the surface of a macrophage upregulates expression of proteins called LMP. These LMP proteins customize proteasomes so that they preferentially cut proteins after hydrophobic or basic amino acids. Why, you ask? Because the TAP transporter and MHC I molecules both favor peptides that have either hydrophobic or basic C-termini. So in antigen presenting cells, LMP proteins modify standard proteasomes so they will produce custom-made peptides, thereby increasing the efficiency of class I display.

Proteasomes are also not too particular about the size of peptides they make, and since the magic number for class I presentation is about nine amino acids, you might imagine that the ER would be flooded with useless peptides that were either too long or too short. However, it turns out that the TAP transporter has the highest affinity for peptides that are between about eight and thirteen amino acids long. Therefore, the TAP transporter screens peptides produced by proteasomes, and preferentially transports those that have the right kinds of C-termini and which are approximately the right length for binding to MHC I molecules.

An important feature of this "chop it up and present it" system is that at least 30% of all newly synthesized proteins are structurally defective (e.g., misfolded) and must be destroyed by proteasomes. Consequently, many proteins are cut up and displayed on class I MHC molecules soon after they are produced. This means that you don't have to wait for proteins to wear out before they can be chopped up and presented, making it possible for the immune system to react more quickly to an infection.

ANTIGEN PRESENTATION BY CLASS II MHC MOLECULES

Whereas class I MHC molecules are designed to present protein fragments to killer T cells, class II MHC molecules present peptides to helper T cells. And in contrast to class I MHC molecules, which are expressed on almost every kind of cell, class II molecules are expressed exclusively on cells of the immune system. This makes sense. Class I molecules specialize in presenting proteins that are manufactured inside the cell,

so the ubiquity of class I molecules gives CTLs a chance to check most cells in the body for viral or other infections. On the other hand, class II MHC molecules function as billboards that advertise what is happening outside the cell to alert helper T cells to danger. Therefore, relatively few cells expressing class II are required for this task – just enough to sample the environment in various parts of the body.

The two proteins that make up the class II MHC molecules (called the α and β chains) are produced in the cytoplasm and are injected into the endoplasmic reticulum where they bind to a third protein, called the invariant chain. This invariant chain protein performs several functions. First, it sits in the groove of the MHC II molecule and keeps it from picking up other peptides in the ER. This is important, because the ER is full of endogenous peptides that have been processed by proteasomes for loading onto class I MHC molecules. If these protein fragments were loaded onto class II molecules, then class I and class II MHC molecules would display the same kind of peptides: those made from proteins produced in the cell. Since the goal is to have class II MHC molecules present antigens that come from outside the cell, the invariant chain performs an important function by acting as a "chaperone" that makes sure "inappropriate suitors" (endogenous peptides) don't get picked up by MHC II molecules in the ER.

The invariant chain's second function is to guide class II MHC molecules out through the Golgi stack to special vesicles in the cytoplasm called "endosomes." It is in these endosomes that class II MHC molecules are loaded with peptides. I have to warn you, however, that when biologists don't understand something very well, they usually call it a "-some" – a suffix that means "body." And this is no exception, because little is known for certain about what goes on in these endosomes.

The current thinking is that while class II MHC molecules are making their way from the ER to the endosome, proteins that are hanging around outside the cell are brought into the cell, enclosed in a phagosome. This phagosome then merges with the endosome, and enzymes present in the endosome chop up the exogenous proteins from the phagosome into peptides. During this time, endosomal enzymes also destroy all of the invariant chain except the piece that is actually guarding the groove of the MHC molecule. Amazingly, although the exogenous proteins and the invariant chain are hacked to pieces by enzymes in the endosome, the class II MHC molecule itself remains unscathed.

Meanwhile, a cellular protein called DM, which also has traveled to the endosome, binds to the MHC molecule and releases the remaining fragment of the invariant chain (called CLIP), allowing an exogenous peptide to be loaded into the now-empty groove of the class II MHC molecule. Finally, the complex of MHC plus peptide is transported to the cell surface for display.

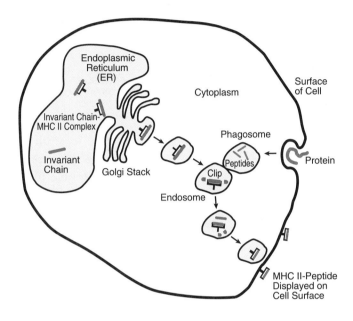

This is probably more or less what happens, but the details are still fuzzy. The important point, however, is that Mother Nature has arranged two separate loading sites and pathways for class I and II MHC molecules. It is this separation of loading sites and pathways that allows the class I billboard to advertise what's going on inside the cell (for killer T cells), and the class II billboard to advertise what's happening outside (for helper T cells).

Although the separation of class I and class II pathways is the rule, under certain experimental conditions, antigens taken up by some antigen presenting cells can end up being presented by class I MHC molecules – violating the "law" that "outside" antigens are presented by class II, but not by class I MHC molecules. Such an unlawful use of the class I display has been termed "cross-presentation." To date, the rules governing cross-presentation have not been clearly defined, and it is not yet known whether, under normal circumstances, cross-presentation occurs with any appreciable frequency in the human body. Consequently, we will have to wait for more experiments to be done to decide whether cross-presentation should be considered to be part of "how the immune system works."

ANTIGEN PRESENTING CELLS

Before a killer T cell can kill or a helper T cell can help, it must be activated. For this to happen, a T cell must recognize its cognate antigen presented by an MHC molecule. But this is not enough. It must also receive a second, co-stimulatory signal. Only certain cells are equipped to provide both class I and class II MHC display and co-stimulation. These are the professional antigen presenting cells (APCs).

Because the job of antigen presenting cells is to activate killer and helper T cells, these cells really should have been named "T cell-activating cells." This would have avoided confusion with the "ordinary" cells in the body, which cannot activate T cells, but which do use class I MHC molecules to "present" antigens made inside these cells to alert killer T cells. To keep this straight, just remember that the term "antigen presenting cell" always refers to those special cells which can provide the high levels of MHC and co-stimulatory molecules required for T cell activation.

Co-stimulation usually involves a protein called B7 on the surface of the antigen presenting cell that "plugs into" a protein called CD28 on the surface of the T cell.

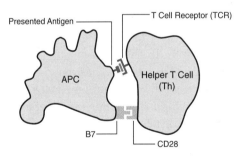

So far, three types of antigen presenting cells have been identified: activated dendritic cells, activated macrophages, and activated B cells. It's interesting that all of these are white blood cells which start life in the bone marrow, migrate out to various sites in the body, and then must be activated before they can function as antigen presenting cells. Because new blood cells are made continuously, APCs can be replenished as needed.

ACTIVATED DENDRITIC CELLS

The story about dendritic cells (DCs) is intriguing, because until just a few years ago, these cells were considered to be only a curiosity. However, it is now appreciated that these once-obscure cells are the most important of all the antigen presenting cells – because dendritic cells can initiate the immune response by activating virgin T cells. Here's how this works.

The first DCs described were starfish-shaped, "Langerhans" cells that are found just below the skin. However, dendritic cells have since been located all over the body. What is now clear is that dendritic cells are "sentinel" cells which take up positions beneath the barriers of epithelial cells that represent our first line of defense. In normal tissues (tissues that have not been infected), dendritic cells are "heavy drinkers" – they take up about four times their volume of extracellular fluid per hour. Mostly, they just take it in and spit it back out. In this "resting" state, DCs express some B7 and relatively low levels of MHC molecules on their surfaces. As a result, resting dendritic cells are not very good at presenting antigen to T cells, especially to virgin T cells, which require extensive receptor crosslinking by MHC-peptide complexes as well as powerful co-stimulation.

If there is a microbial invasion, and the tissues in which the dendritic cell resides become a battle site, the lifestyle of this heavy drinker changes dramatically, because the dendritic cell becomes "activated." This occurs when receptors on the surface of the DC recognize molecules that are characteristic of a microbial invader (e.g., LPS from Gram-negative bacteria) or battle cytokines, which signal that the innate system is engaged in a struggle. For example, when TNF secreted by battling macrophages binds to receptors on the surface of a dendritic cell, phagocytosis ceases, and something magic happens – the DC leaves the tissues and migrates through the lymphatic system to the nearest lymph node. It is this ability to "travel when stimulated by battle signals" that makes the dendritic antigen presenting cell so special.

Inside a resting dendritic cell are large numbers of class II MHC molecules just waiting to be loaded. When the resting DC is activated, these "reserve" class II MHC molecules are loaded with antigens from the battle scene. And by the time the DC reaches its destination, these battle antigen-loaded class II MHC molecules are displayed on the surface of the dendritic cell. Also during its journey, the DC upregulates expression of class I MHC molecules. Consequently, if the dendritic cell was infected by viruses or other parasites at the battle scene, fragments of proteins made by these infecting parasites can be efficiently presented in the

lymph node by class I MHC molecules. Finally, while traveling, the dendritic cell increases production of B7 co-stimulatory proteins. So by the time it reaches a lymph node, the traveling dendritic cell has everything it needs to activate virgin T cells – high levels of class I and class II MHC molecules and plenty of B7 proteins.

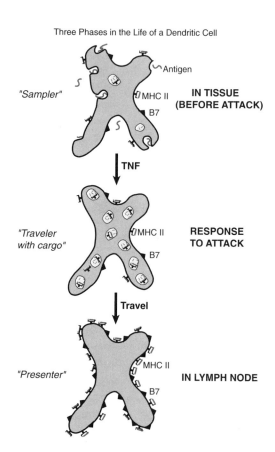

Three Phases in the Life of a Dendritic Cell

Now, why do you think it would be a good idea to have DCs, which wildly sample antigens out in the tissues, stop sampling when they begin their journey to a lymph node? Of course. Dendritic cells take a "snapshot" of what is happening on the "front lines," and carry this image to the lymph node. There they activate virgin T cells whose T cell receptors recognize the invader that is "in the picture." Since lymph nodes are "dating bars" where T cells hang out, the traveling dendritic cells actually bring the antigen from the battle to the place where virgin T cells are located. The fact that battle cytokines such as TNF trigger the migration of DCs to a lymph node also makes perfect sense. After all, you want DCs to travel and present antigen only if a battle is on.

When our Defense Department reacts to a threat

to our national security, it follows the "principle of proportional response." For instance, if Iranian terrorists were to fire on one of our embassies, we wouldn't start dropping atom bombs on Iran. No, we would respond in a way that was more appropriate to such a limited threat. Likewise, it is important that the magnitude of an immune response be in proportion to the seriousness of the attack. Fortunately, the system is designed to make this happen. Let me explain.

Dendritic cells only travel to nearby lymph nodes when they are activated by battle cytokines. If the infection is serious, many battle cytokines will be produced, and many dendritic cells will set off on this journey. In addition, before they leave the tissues, dendritic cells produce special cytokines (called chemokines) that influence precursor cells (monocytes) to leave the blood, enter the tissues, and become dendritic cells. So activated dendritic cells recruit their own replacements. These newly arrived dendritic cells can then be activated and dispatched to lymph nodes to amplify the response to the invasion. On the other hand, if the attack is relatively mild, fewer battle cytokines will be produced, correspondingly fewer dendritic cells will travel, and fewer replacements will be recruited. Now, because the number of B and T cells that become activated in lymph nodes will depend on the number of dendritic cells that bring "news" of the battle, the system is set up so that the "punishment fits the crime": The magnitude of the immune response will depend on the severity of the infection.

Once an activated (immunologists usually call them "mature") DC reaches a lymph node, it only lives for a few days. This short lifetime may seem strange at first. After all, a few days doesn't give a dendritic cell very long to meet up with a virgin T cell that is circulating through the lymph nodes looking for its cognate antigen. However, this short "presentation" life insures that the snapshot of the battle which is carried by the dendritic cell is up-to-date. Indeed, because dendritic cells recruit their own replacements, if the battle continues, more DCs can be activated to carry fresh images of the battle into the lymph nodes. In addition, when the invader has been subdued and DCs stop traveling, the short lifetime of mature dendritic cells makes it easier to turn the immune system back off.

So dendritic antigen presenting cells are sentinel cells that "sample" antigens out in the tissues. If there is an invasion, DCs become activated and travel to nearby lymph nodes. There they initiate the adaptive immune response by presenting antigens collected at the battle scene to virgin T cells. Activated DCs are short lived, and the rapid turnover of dendritic cells ensures that the "pictures" they bring to the lymph node are continually updated. Moreover, the number of dendritic cells dispatched from the tissues and the number of replacement dendritic cells recruited will depend on the severity of the attack. Consequently, the immune system is able to mount a response that is proportional to the danger posed by the invasion. Can you imagine a more ingenious system for antigen presentation? I don't think so!

ACTIVATED MACROPHAGES

Macrophages are also sentinel cells that stand guard over those areas of our bodies that are exposed to the outside world. They are very adaptable cells that can function as garbage collectors, antigen presenting cells, or ferocious killers, depending on the signals they receive from the microenvironment in which they reside. In a resting state, macrophages are good at tidying up, but they are not much good at antigen presentation. This is because macrophages only express enough MHC and co-stimulatory molecules to function as antigen presenting cells after they have been activated by battle cytokines such as IFN-γ.

So like dendritic cells, macrophages efficiently present antigen only when there is something dangerous that is worth presenting. Unlike DCs, however, macrophages don't travel. Whereas DCs can be pictured as "photojournalists" who take snapshots and then leave the battlefield to file their stories, macrophages are like soldiers who must stand and fight. After all, macrophages are one of our main weapons in the early defense against invaders. This lack of mobility raises an interesting question: What good is the activated macrophage's ability to present antigen if it can't travel to lymph nodes where the virgin T cells are located?

Once they have been activated by dendritic cells, T cells exit the lymph nodes and enter inflamed tissues to help with the battle. However, these activated T cells must be continuously re-stimulated, otherwise they think the battle has been won, and they go back to a resting state or die of neglect. That's where the activated macrophage comes into play. These cells act as "refueling stations" out in the tissues by keeping experienced T cells activated so they can continue to participate in the battle. So dendritic antigen presenting cells activate virgin T cells in lymph nodes, whereas out at the battle scene, activated macrophages mainly function to re-stimulate experienced T cells.

ACTIVATED B CELLS

The third professional APC is the activated B cell. A virgin B cell is not much good at antigen presentation because it expresses only low levels of class II MHC molecules and little or no B7. However, once a B cell has been activated, the levels of class II MHC molecules and B7 proteins on its surface increase dramatically. As a result, an <u>experienced</u> B cell is able to act as an antigen presenting cell for Th cells. The current thinking is that B cells are not used as APCs during the initial stages of an infection, because at that time they are still naive – they haven't been activated. However, later in the course of the infection or during subsequent infections, presentation of antigen by experienced B cells plays an important role. Indeed, B cells have one great advantage over the other APCs – B cells can concentrate antigen for presentation. Here's how this works.

After a B cell's receptors have bound to their cognate antigen, the whole complex of BCR plus antigen is removed from the cell surface and dragged into the cell. Once inside, the antigen is processed, loaded onto class II MHC molecules, and transported back to the cell surface for presentation.

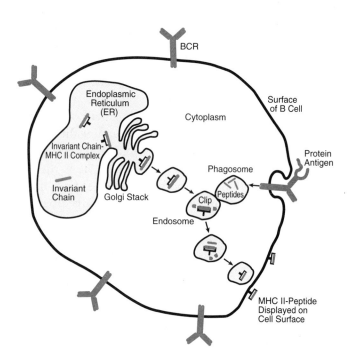

Because BCRs have such a high affinity for antigen, these receptors act like "magnets," collecting antigen for presentation to Th cells. Since a threshold number of T cell receptors must be crosslinked by presented antigen before a Th cell can be activated, it is estimated that B cells have a 100- to 10,000-fold advantage over other APCs in activating helper T cells at times when there is relatively little antigen around. Presentation of antigen by B cells is also very fast. Less than half an hour elapses between the time antigen is captured by a B cell's receptors and the time it is displayed on the cell surface by class II MHC molecules.

In summary, when an invader is first encountered, all the B cells that could recognize that invader are virgins, so the important APCs are activated dendritic cells. Then, while the battle is raging, activated macrophages out at the "front" present antigen to warring T cells to keep them "pumped up." Later, if this same invader is encountered again, experienced memory B cells left over from the first attack are the most important APCs – because they can get the adaptive immune response cranked up quickly by concentrating small amounts of antigen for presentation.

THE LOGIC OF MHC PRESENTATION

To really appreciate why antigen presentation is one of Mother Nature's greatest inventions, we need to think a little about the logic behind this amazing activity. For starters, we need to ask the question: Why bother with MHC presentation at all? Why not just let a T cell's receptors recognize unpresented antigen the way a B cell's receptors do? This is really a two-part question, since we are talking about two rather different displays: class I and class II. So let's discuss these displays one at a time.

Certainly one reason for class I presentation is to focus the attention of killer T cells on infected cells, not on viruses and other pathogens that are outside our cells in blood and tissues. So long as pathogens remain outside of cells, antibodies can tag them for destruction by professional phagocytes, and can bind to them to prevent them from initiating an infection. Since each plasma B cell can pump out about 10,000 antibody molecules per second, these antibodies are "cheap" weapons that deal quite effectively with extracellular invaders. However, once microbes enter a cell, antibodies can't get at them. So killer T cells are "expensive," high-tech weapons specifically designed to deal with infected cells – and the requirement that killer T cells recognize antigens presented by class I MHC molecules on infected cells insures that CTLs won't waste their time going after invaders while they are outside of cells.

In addition, it would be extremely dangerous to have unpresented antigen signal T cell killing. Imagine how terrible it would be if uninfected cells happened to have debris from dead viruses stuck to their surfaces, and killer T cells recognized this unpresented antigen and killed these "innocent bystander" cells. That certainly wouldn't do.

There's another reason why class I display is so important. Most proteins made in a pathogen-infected cell remain inside the cell, and never make their way to the cell surface. So without class I display, pathogen-infected cells could go undetected. In fact, part of the magic of the class I MHC display is that, in principle, every protein of an invading pathogen can be chopped up and displayed by class I MHC molecules.

Finally, because their receptors recognize "native" antigens that have not been fragmented and presented, B cells are actually at a disadvantage. The reason is that most proteins must be folded in order to function properly. As a result of this folding, many targets (epitopes) that a B cell's receptors might recognize are unavailable for viewing, because they are on the inside of a folded protein molecule. In contrast, when a protein is chopped up into short pieces and presented by class I MHC molecules, epitopes cannot be hidden from killer T cells.

So class I MHC presentation makes a lot of sense, but what about class II presentation? Couldn't helper T cells just recognize unpresented antigen? After all, they aren't killers, so there isn't the problem of bystander killing. That's true, of course, but there is still a safety issue here. Because antigen presenting cells only present antigen efficiently when a battle is going on, both the helper T cell and the antigen presenting cell must "agree" that there is a problem before a helper T cell can be activated. By requiring that helper T cells only recognize presented antigen, Mother Nature guarantees that the decision to deploy the deadly adaptive immune system is not made by a single cell.

Also, like class I molecules, class II molecules present small fragments of proteins. As a result, the number of targets that a helper T cell can "see" during presentation far exceeds those available for viewing in a large, folded protein. The consequence of this expanded number of targets is a stronger and more diverse immune reaction in which many different helper T cells will be activated whose receptors recognize different epitopes present on the antigens of each invader.

So having MHC molecules present antigen makes good sense. But why did Mother Nature make MHC molecules so polymorphic? After all, there are so many different forms in the human population that most of us inherit genes for six different class I molecules. Doesn't this seem a bit excessive? I mean, why not just let everybody express the same MHC I molecule?

Well, suppose we all did have just one gene for class I MHC proteins, and that it was the same for everyone. Now imagine that a virus mutated so that none of its peptides would bind to that single MHC I molecule. Such a virus could wipe out the entire human population, because no killer T cells could be activated to destroy virus-infected cells. So polymorphic MHC molecules give at least some people in the population a chance of surviving an attack by a clever pathogen. Moreover, the fact that each of us has the possibility of "owning" up to six different class I MHC molecules increases the probability that each of us will have at least one class I MHC molecule into which a given pathogen's protein fragments will fit. Indeed, recent studies have shown that on average, AIDS patients who have inherited the maximum number of different class I MHC molecules (six) live significantly longer than patients who have genes for only five or fewer different class I molecules. The thinking here is that as the AIDS virus mutates, having a larger number of different class I molecules increases the probability that mutated viral proteins can be presented.

Okay, so if having six MHC I molecules is good, wouldn't 1,000 be better? Why not 10,000? After all, Mother Nature certainly could have arranged to make our MHC molecules as diverse as the B and T cell receptors, just by using the strategy of mixing and matching gene segments. But she didn't do this – and for a very good reason.

Let's imagine that some "superhuman" had 1,000 different class I MHC molecules instead of the six we actually have. Because a T cell's receptors must recognize not only the presented peptide, but also the particular MHC molecule that is doing the presenting (more about this "dual recognition" in the next lecture), each of the superhuman's T cells would only be trained to recognize peptides presented by one of his 1,000 MHC molecules. Now, on your average antigen presenting cell, there are only about 100,000 MHC molecules. Consequently, the T cell receptors on each of the superhuman's T cells would only recognize about 100 of these molecules. And for a virgin T cell to be activated, about 100 of its T cell receptors must recognize a particular MHC/peptide combination. So if each type of MHC molecule on the super-human's antigen presenting cells presented more than one antigen (and MHC molecules generally present thousands), there would be too few of any one kind of MHC molecule presenting a given antigen to activate any of his T cells. In such a case, the "superhuman" would probably end up as a "dead human," because he would have no activated T cells. There are some subtleties here that would keep the situation from being quite this bad, but you get the idea: With 1,000 different MHC molecules, the display would be too "dilute" to efficiently activate T cells. No, I don't know why she picked six. I guess it must have been a good compromise.

In summary, antigen presentation by MHC molecules is an elegant solution to a number of problems that face the immune system: Presentation by class I MHC molecules ensures that killer T cells stay focused on infected cells, that innocent bystanders are not killed by mistake, and that a clever pathogen cannot hide in an infected cell by keeping all its proteins internal. MHC presentation of protein fragments greatly increases the universe of antigens that are available for killer T cells and helper T cells to recognize, because epitopes hidden in a folded protein are revealed. And because MHC molecules are so polymorphic, it is likely that at least some humans will have MHC molecules which can display protein fragments from any pathogen. Finally (and perhaps most importantly), helper T cells and killer T cells must recognize their cognate antigens presented by antigen presenting cells before they can be activated. This requirement for antigen presentation during activation sets up a fail-safe system in which the decision to activate the adaptive immune system is never made by a single cell.

MHC PROTEINS AND ORGAN TRANSPLANTS

In addition to their "natural" role in antigen presentation, MHC molecules also are important in the "unnatural" setting of organ and tissue transplantation. Transplantation studies actually began in the 1930s with experiments involving mouse tumors. In those days, tumors were usually induced by rubbing some horrible chemical on the skin of a mouse, and then waiting for a long time for a tumor to develop. Because it was so much trouble to make these tumors, biologists wanted to keep the tumor cells alive for study after the mouse had died. They did this by injecting some of the tumor cells into another, healthy mouse, where the cells would continue to grow. What they observed, however, was

that the tumor cells could only be successfully transplanted when the two mice were from a strain of mice in which there had been a lot of inbreeding. And the more inbred the strain, the better the chance for survival of the transplant. This provided the impetus for the creation of a number of inbred mouse strains that immunologists depend on today. Just so you know, it takes over two years of constant breeding to produce a strain of mice that is truly inbred – a strain in which all the mice have essentially the same genetic makeup.

Once inbred mouse strains were available, immunologists began to study the transplantation of normal tissues from one mouse to another. Right away they noticed that if a small patch of skin from one mouse (the donor) was grafted onto the skin of another mouse, this new skin retained its healthy pink color and continued to grow so long as the two mice were from the same inbred strain. In contrast, when this experiment was tried with mice that were not inbred, the transplanted skin turned white within hours (suggesting the blood supply had been cut off) and invariably died. Immunologists figured this immediate graft rejection must be due to some genetic incompatibility, because it did not occur with inbred mice that have the same genes. To identify the genes that are involved in "tissue compatibility" (histocompatibility), immunologists bred mice to create strains that differed by only a few genes, yet which were still incompatible for tissue transplants. Whenever they did these experiments, they kept identifying genes that were grouped in a complex on mouse chromosome seventeen – a complex they eventually called the "major histocompatibility complex" or MHC.

So the MHC molecules that we have been discussing in the context of antigen presentation are the very same molecules that are responsible for immediate rejection of transplanted organs. It turns out that killer T cells are particularly sensitive to MHC molecules that are "foreign," and when they see them, they attack and kill the cells that express them. One of their favorite targets are the cells that make up the blood vessels contained within the donated organ. By destroying these vessels, CTLs cut off the blood supply to the transplanted organ, usually resulting in its death. It is for this reason that transplant surgeons try to match donors and recipients that have the same MHC molecules. However, finding such a match is difficult. Indeed, it is estimated that if you had access to a bank of bone marrow contributed by 10,000 different individuals who were not related to you, the chances of your finding a match to your class I MHC molecules would only be about 70%. So the diversity of MHC molecules that is so important in protecting us from new invaders creates a real problem for organ transplantation. Perhaps if Mother Nature had known that we would be swapping organs around, she might not have made MHC molecules quite so polymorphic!

SUMMARY FIGURE

Now that you understand how antigens are presented and why presentation by class I and class II MHC molecules is such a great idea, we need to turn our attention to the cells that are "looking at" these two kinds of display – the helper T cell and the CTL. How these cells react to presented antigen is the subject of our next lecture.

You will notice that our summary figure now includes antigen presenting cells with their MHC and B7 molecules.

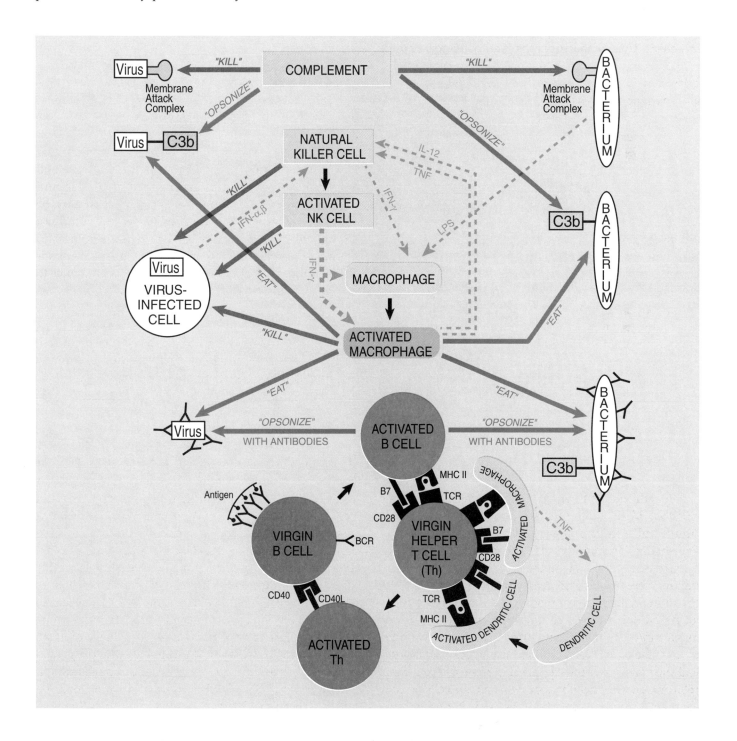

THOUGHT QUESTIONS

1. Mother Nature uses "failsafe technology" to prevent inappropriate activation of the immune system. Can you give several examples of this strategy?

2. Give several reasons why antigen presentation by class I MHC molecules is important for the function of the adaptive immune system.

3. Why does antigen presentation by class II MHC molecules make good sense?

4. Describe the different roles that activated dendritic cells, activated macrophages, and activated B cells play in the presentation of antigen during the course of an infection.

5. During their lifetimes, dendritic antigen presenting cells can be "samplers," "travelers," and "presenters." Describe what DCs are doing during each of these three stages.

6. Some peptides are presented more efficiently than others. What factors influence the efficiency of presentation by class I and class II MHC molecules?

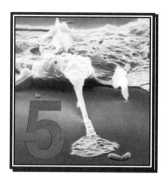

T CELLS AND CYTOKINES

REVIEW

In the last lecture we talked about MHC molecules and antigen presenting cells (APCs). Class I MHC molecules function as billboards that display what is going on inside a cell. For example, when a virus infects a cell, it uses that cell's biosynthetic machinery to produce viral proteins. Some of these proteins are cut up into small pieces (peptides) by the proteasome, and carried by the TAP transporters into the endoplasmic reticulum (ER). There the peptides are "interviewed" by class I molecules. Those that are about nine amino acids in length with appropriate amino acids at their ends are bound in the grooves of class I MHC molecules, and are transported to the surface of the cell. By scanning the MHC I-peptide complexes displayed there, killer T cells can "look into a cell" to determine whether it has been infected and should be destroyed.

Class II MHC molecules are also billboards, but they are designed to alert helper T cells that a battle is being waged. Class II molecules are assembled in the ER, just like class I molecules, but because invariant chain proteins occupy their binding grooves, class II molecules do not pick up peptides in the ER. Instead, the class II–invariant chain complex is transported out of the ER and into another cellular compartment called an endosome. There they meet up with proteins that have been taken into the cell by phagocytosis and cut up into peptides by enzymes. These peptides then replace the invariant chains that have been guarding the grooves of the class II molecules, and the MHC-peptide complexes are transported to the cell surface for display to Th cells. By this clever mechanism, class II molecules pick up peptides derived from proteins taken in from outside the cell, but avoid peptides derived from proteins made within the cell.

The display by MHC molecules of fragmented proteins has several advantages over a display of intact proteins. First, most viral proteins normally remain inside the infected cell and are not found on the cell surface. So these proteins would never be seen by killer T cells unless they were advertised by class I MHC molecules. In addition, because protein folding can hide large portions of a protein from view, chopping a protein up into small peptides reveals many potential T cell targets that would be inaccessible in an intact protein. All in all, MHC display is a wonderful idea, because it greatly increases the probability that CTLs will recognize an infected cell and that helper T cells will be alerted to a microbial attack.

Before killer T cells or helper T cells can function, they must be activated, and it is the task of the antigen presenting cell to do this activation. The requirement for activation insures that T cells only spring into action when both the T cell and the antigen presenting cell agree that there has been an invasion. In addition to expressing class I and class II molecules, APCs also provide the co-stimulatory signals required for T cell activation. The most important antigen presenting cell during the initial stages of an attack is the dendritic cell, because this cell can activate virgin T cells. When this amazing cell is activated by "danger signals," it migrates with its cargo of "battle antigen" to a nearby lymph node. There, the dendritic cell uses class II MHC molecules to display fragments of proteins it has collected out in the tissues, and class I MHC molecules to display fragments of proteins made by viruses or other parasites that have infected the dendritic cell out at the battle site. In this way, the dendritic cell effectively takes a snapshot of what is going on in the battle zone, carries it to the place where T cells are plentiful, and then does its "show and tell" thing to activate these T cells.

Macrophages, activated by danger signals, can also function as antigen presenting cells. However, activated macrophages don't travel to lymph nodes to present antigen – they stay put in the tissues and battle the invaders. Consequently, macrophages aren't very useful for activating naive T cells, because virgin T cells are not found out in the tissues. The antigen presenting function of macrophages comes into play after the adaptive immune system has been activated, at a time when "experienced" T cells enter the tissues to help or kill. There, antigen presented by activated macrophages can keep the experienced T cells fired up, prolonging the time that they are effective in dealing with invaders.

Activated B cells are the third type of antigen presenting cell, but again, these cells aren't useful in initiating the adaptive response. The reason is that before B cells can function as antigen presenting cells, they must first be activated by helper T cells – and Th cells must wait to be activated by dendritic cells. So B cells don't get "certified" to be antigen presenting cells until after the adaptive immune response has fired up. However, once activated, B cells have a great advantage over dendritic cells and macrophages: B cells can use their receptors as "antigen collectors" to concentrate small amounts of antigen for presentation. Consequently, relatively late in the initial infection or early in a subsequent infection by the same attacker, B cells play a major role as antigen presenting cells.

T CELLS AND CYTOKINES

In this lecture, we're going to focus on T cells – how they are activated and what they do. To begin, let's talk about T cell receptors (TCRs) – those molecules on the surface of the T cell that function as the cell's "eyes" on the world. Without these receptors, T cells would be flying blind with no way to sense what's going on outside.

T CELL RECEPTORS

T cell receptors come in two flavors: $\alpha\beta$ and $\gamma\delta$. Each type of receptor is composed of two proteins, either α and β or γ and δ. Like the heavy and light chains of the B cell receptor, the genes for α, β, γ, and δ are assembled by mixing and matching gene segments. In fact, in T and B cells, the same proteins (RAG1 and RAG2) initiate the splicing of gene segments by making double-stranded breaks in chromosomal DNA. As the gene segments are mixed and matched, a "competition" ensues from which each T cell emerges with either an $\alpha\beta$ or a $\gamma\delta$ receptor, but not both. Generally, all the TCRs on a mature T cell are identical – although there are exceptions to this rule.

Over 95% of the T cells in circulation have $\alpha\beta$ T cell receptors and express either a CD4 or CD8 "co-receptor" molecule in addition to the $\alpha\beta$ proteins. In contrast, most $\gamma\delta$ T cells do not express either CD4 or CD8. T cells with $\gamma\delta$ receptors are most abundant in areas like the intestine, the uterus, and the tongue, which are in contact with the outside world. Interestingly, mice have lots of $\gamma\delta$ T cells in the epidermal layer of their skin, but humans do not. This serves to remind us that so far as the immune system is concerned, humans are not just big mice.

Although $\alpha\beta$ TCRs are thought to be about as diverse as BCRs, $\gamma\delta$ receptors are much less diverse. For example, the receptors of $\gamma\delta$ T cells in the tongue and uterus tend to favor certain gene segments during rearrangement, whereas $\gamma\delta$ receptors in the intestine prefer other combinations of gene segments. The thinking here is that, like players on the innate immune system team, $\gamma\delta$ T cells stand watch on the "front lines," and have receptors that are "tuned" to recognize invaders that commonly enter at certain locations.

There is a lot about $\gamma\delta$ T cells that is still mysterious. For example, it is not known where these cells are educated. T cells with $\alpha\beta$ receptors are taught in the thymus not to react against our own self peptides. Although $\gamma\delta$ T cells are also found in the thymus, nude mice, which lack a functional thymus, still produce $\gamma\delta$ T cells. In most cases it is also not known exactly what $\gamma\delta$ T cells recognize, but it is believed that, like B cells, $\gamma\delta$ T cells focus on unpresented antigen. Finally, the exact function of $\gamma\delta$ T cells is not clear, although some of them appear to kill cells that become "stressed" as the result of a microbial infection.

Because much more is known about T cells with

αβ receptors, we will focus on these cells for the remainder of this lecture. The αβ receptors recognize a complex between a peptide and an MHC molecule on the surface of a cell. What I mean by "MHC-peptide complex" is a peptide bound in the groove of an MHC molecule. I use the word "complex" to emphasize the fact that the TCR recognizes both the peptide and the MHC molecule. A given T cell will have receptors that recognize peptides associated with class I MHC molecules or with class II MHC molecules, but not both.

HOW A T CELL'S RECEPTORS SIGNAL

Once a TCR has recognized its cognate antigen presented by an MHC molecule, the next step is to transmit a signal from the surface of the T cell, where recognition takes place, to the nucleus of the T cell. The idea is that for the T cell to switch from a resting state to a state of activation, gene expression must be altered, and these genes are, of course, located in the cell's nucleus. Normally, this type of signaling across the cell membrane involves a transmembrane protein that has two parts: an external region which binds to a molecule (called a ligand) that is outside the cell, plus an internal region that initiates a biochemical cascade which conveys the "ligand bound" signal to the nucleus. Here the TCR runs into a bit of a problem. As is true of the BCR, the αβ TCR has a perfectly fine extracellular domain that can bind to its ligand (the combination of MHC molecule and peptide), but the cytoplasmic tails of the α and β proteins are only about three amino acids long – way too short to signal.

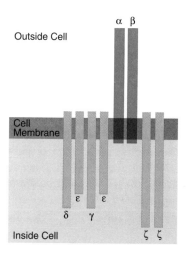

To handle the signaling part, Mother Nature had to add a few bells and whistles to the TCR: a complex of proteins collectively called CD3. In humans, this signaling complex is made up of four different proteins: γ, δ, ε, and ζ (gamma, delta, epsilon, and zeta). Please note, however, that the ζ and δ proteins that are part of the CD3 complex are not the same as the γ and δ proteins that make up the γδ T cell receptor. The CD3 proteins are anchored in the cell membrane, and have cytoplasmic tails that are long enough to signal just fine. As with BCRs, signaling by TCRs involves clustering these receptors together in one area of the T cell surface. When this happens, a threshold number of kinase enzymes is recruited by the cytoplasmic tails of the CD3 proteins, and the activation signal is dispatched to the nucleus.

Although the details about how this signaling works are still somewhat sketchy, there are some interesting points about this six-protein, T cell receptor. First, the whole complex of proteins (α, β, γ, δ, ε, ζ) is transported to the cell surface as a unit. If any one of these proteins fails to be made, you don't get a TCR on the surface. So most immunologists consider the functional, mature TCR to be this whole complex of proteins. After all, the α and β proteins are great for recognition, but they can't signal. And together, the γ, δ, ε, and ζ proteins signal just fine, but they are totally blind to what's going on outside the cell. You need both parts to make it work.

Back when the α and β chains of the TCR were first discovered, it was thought that the TCR was just an on/off switch whose only function was to signal activation. But now that you have heard about the CD3 proteins, let me ask you: Does this look like a simple on/off switch? No way. Mother Nature certainly wouldn't make an on/off switch with six proteins! No, this TCR is quite versatile. It can send signals that result in very different outcomes, depending on how, when, and where it is triggered. For example, during their education in the thymus, T cell receptors are used to trigger suicide (death by apoptosis) if the TCR recognizes MHC plus self peptides. Later, if its TCRs recognize their cognate antigen presented by MHC molecules, but the T cell does not receive the required co-stimulatory signals, that T cell is neutered (anergized) so it can't function. And, of course, when a TCR is engaged by cognate antigen and co-stimulatory signals are available, the TCR signals activation. So this same T cell receptor, depending on the situation, signals death, anergy, or activation. In fact, there are now documented cases in which the alteration of a single amino acid in a presented peptide can change the signal from activation to death! Clearly this is no on/off switch, and immunologists are working very hard to understand exactly how TCR signaling is "wired," and what factors influence the signaling outcome.

CD4 AND CD8 CO-RECEPTORS

Doesn't it seem that Mother Nature got carried away with the CD4 and CD8 co-receptors? I mean, there are two proteins, α and β, to use for antigen recognition; and four more, γ, δ, ε, and ζ, to use for signaling. Wouldn't you think that would do it? Apparently not, so there must be essential features of the system that require CD4 and CD8 co-receptors. Let's see what these might be.

Killer T cells and helper T cells perform two very different functions, and they "look at" two different molecules, class I or class II MHC, respectively, to get their cues. But how do CTLs know to focus on peptides presented by class I molecules – and how do Th cells know to scan APCs for peptides presented by class II? After all, it wouldn't be so great if a CTL got confused, recognized a class II-peptide complex on an APC, and killed the antigen presenting cell! So here's where CD4 and CD8 come in. CTLs generally express CD8 and Th cells usually express CD4. These co-receptor molecules are designed to clip onto either class I MHC (CD8) or class II MHC molecules (CD4).

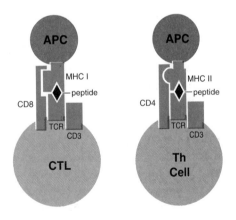

These "clips" strengthen the adhesion between the T cell and the APC, so CD4 and CD8 co-receptors function to focus the attention of CTLs and Th cells on the proper MHC molecule. But there is more to the story, because it turns out that CD4 and CD8 are signaling

molecules just like the CD3 complex of proteins. Both CD4 and CD8 have tails that extend through the cell wall and into the interior (cytoplasm) of the cell, and both of these tails have the right characteristics to signal. In addition, because CD4 is a single protein and CD8 is composed of two different proteins, the signals that these co-receptors send are likely to be quite different – perhaps as different as "help" and "kill." In contrast to CD3 molecules, which are glued rather tightly to the αβ T cell receptor on the cell surface, the CD4 and CD8 co-receptors usually are only loosely associated with the TCR/CD3 proteins. The latest thinking is that once the TCR engages its cognate antigen presented by the MHC molecule, the CD4 or CD8 co-receptors then clip on and stabilize the TCR-MHC-peptide interaction, thereby strengthening the signal sent by the TCR.

When T cells begin maturing in the thymus, they express both types of co-receptors on their surfaces. Immunologists call them CD4+CD8+ cells. Then, as they mature, expression of one or the other of these co-receptors is downregulated, and a cell becomes either CD4+ or CD8+. So how does a given T cell decide whether it will express CD4 or CD8 when it grows up? Well, immunologists are not any more certain about how T cells decide to be CD4+ or CD8+ than they are about how B cells decide to be plasma cells or memory cells. Some think that it is just a random process in which T cells downregulate expression of one type of co-receptor. Others propose that if a TCR happens to bind, say, to a class I molecule on the surface of a cell in the thymus, a signal is sent to downregulate CD4 expression (the "instructive" model). Although recent experiments favor the instructive model, other experimental results argue against it – so the question of how T cells "pick" their co-receptor molecules is still unanswered.

CO-STIMULATION

In naive T cells, the "connection" between the T cell's receptors and the cell's nucleus is not very good. It's as if the T cell had an electrical system in which a large resistor were placed between the sensor (the TCR) and the piece of equipment it is designed to regulate (gene expression in the nucleus). Because of this "resistor," a lot of the signal from the TCR is lost as it travels to the nucleus. The result is that a prohibitively large number of TCRs would have to engage their cognate antigen before the signal that reaches the nucleus would be strong enough to have any effect. If, however, while the TCRs are engaged, the T cell also receives co-stimulation, the signal from the TCRs is amplified many times, so that fewer (probably about 100-fold fewer) TCRs must be engaged to activate a naive T cell. So in addition to having their T cell receptors ligated by MHC-peptide, naive T cells must also receive co-stimulatory signals before they can be activated. Co-stimulation can be thought of as an "amplifier" that strengthens the "I'm engaged" signal sent by the T cell's receptors, thereby lowering the threshold number of TCRs that must be crosslinked by MHC-peptide complexes.

Interestingly, once a naive T cell has been activated, the connection between the TCRs and the nucleus strengthens. It is as if experienced T cells are "re-wired" so that the resistors present in naive T cells are bypassed. As a result of this re-wiring, in an "experienced" T cell, amplification of the TCR signal is not as important as it is in virgin T cells. Consequently, experienced T cells have a reduced requirement for co-stimulation. Recent experiments have suggested a mechanism by which co-stimulation might amplify the TCR signal. Here's how this is thought to work.

Although it is easy to visualize the surface of a cell as a rigid covering, the fact is that the plasma membrane that cloaks a human cell is more like a viscous fluid than a rigid shell. Indeed, proteins that are on the cell surface "float" around fairly freely in this oily gunk. Importantly, the composition of the cell membrane is not homogeneous, and certain proteins and certain types of lipid molecules form aggregates called "rafts." When immunologists examined these cholesterol-rich rafts, they found that they contained a large number of the "downstream" signaling molecules that are used to carry the "TCR engaged" signal from the cell surface to the nucleus. Immunologists also found that before a naive T cell is activated, most of its T cell receptors are not associated with these rafts. However, once a T cell's receptors engage their cognate antigen, the TCRs and the rafts come together. This brings the TCRs into close contact with the downstream signaling molecules, and that completes the circuit to the nucleus.

It also turns out that before naive T cells are activated, they don't have many of these lipid rafts on their surfaces. Most of them are stored inside the cell as parts of other membranous structures. And it is this dearth of rafts on the cell surface that is thought to be the reason the connection between TCRs and the nucleus in a virgin T cell is not a good one – there just aren't enough wires (downstream signaling molecules) available to efficiently carry the signal. However, if a virgin T cell's receptors engage their cognate antigen <u>and</u> appropriate co-stimulation is supplied by the antigen presenting cell, the lipid rafts that are stored inside the cell are rushed to the surface. Now the signal from the TCR can be carried by the additional downstream signaling molecules associated with these rafts, and a strong signal can be sent to the nucleus.

So it is believed that the key to signal amplification by co-stimulation is that co-stimulation recruits lipid rafts to the surface of the T cell. Consistent with this model, experienced T cells have many more rafts on their surfaces than do naive cells. So, as you'd predict, re-activation of experienced T cells doesn't require the strong co-stimulation needed initially to activate virgin T cells – the rafts in experienced T cells are already on the surface, just waiting to carry the signal.

Although a number of different molecules have been identified that can co-stimulate T cells, certainly the best studied examples are the B7 proteins (B7-1 and B7-2), which are expressed on the surface of antigen presenting cells. B7 molecules provide co-stimulation to T cells by plugging into receptors on the T cell surface. So far, two of these receptors have been identified: CD28 and CTLA-4. Most T cells express CD28 proteins, but CTLA-4 molecules are only expressed after a T cell has been activated. The current thinking is that B7 proteins on APCs ligate the CD28 receptors on virgin T cells, thereby providing the co-stimulatory signal necessary for activation. Then, once the cell has been activated, ligation of CTLA-4 receptors by B7 proteins helps to turn off or "deactivate" the T cell. Turning off the adaptive immune response once its job is done is very important. Otherwise, we'd fill up with activated B and T cells that could protect us against enemies past, but not against present or future invaders. Using CTLA-4 ligation as a negative regulator of T cell activation seems to be one way this is accomplished.

A TIME-LAPSE PHOTO OF HELPER T CELL ACTIVATION

I'll bet your picture of helper T cell activation is that dendritic cells in the lymph nodes flit from naive T cell to naive T cell, activating them. This certainly used to be how I visualized the process. It turns out, however, that activation of a naive helper T cell actually takes hours. Exactly how many hours is still controversial, but it is clear that "flitting about" is not what dendritic cells do.

During the hours required to activate a naive T cell, a number of important events take place. First, adhesion molecules on the surface of the dendritic cell bind to their adhesion partners on the T cell, bringing the two cells together. This Velcro-like interaction is nonspecific and not very strong, but it does give the helper cell's TCRs a chance to scan the MHC-peptide complexes on the surface of the APC. If the TCRs do not see their cognate antigen on the dendritic cell's billboard, the cells part, and the Th cell goes on to scan other APCs.

If, however, a helper T cell's TCRs do find their match, the CD4 co-receptor molecules on the surface of the T cell clip onto the class II MHC molecules on the dendritic cell and strengthen the interaction between the two cells. In addition, the engagement of its TCRs upregulates the expression of adhesion molecules on the Th cell surface, so that more adhesion molecules connect, strengthening the "glue" that holds the APC and the T cell together. This is important, because the binding between a TCR and an MHC-peptide complex is actually rather weak. In fact, the ability to express the adhesion molecules required to keep APCs and T cells together long enough for a threshold level of TCR engagement to be reached is one feature that sets APCs apart from "ordinary" cells. The "clustering" of TCRs and adhesion molecules at the point of contact between the APC and the T cell results in the formation of what immunologists call an "immunological synapse."

Engagement of a helper T cell's receptors also upregulates expression of CD40L proteins on the surface of the T cell. When these proteins plug into the CD40 proteins on the surface of the dendritic cell, several remarkable things happen. Although dendritic cells enter lymph nodes in a "mature state" in which they express MHC and co-stimulatory molecules (e.g., B7), the expression level of these proteins increases when the CD40 protein on the APC is engaged by the CD40L protein on the T cell. Engagement of a dendritic cell's CD40 proteins also can cause the cell to secrete cytokines (e.g., IL-12), and can prolong the life of the dendritic cell. This extension of a "useful" dendritic cell's life span makes perfect sense. It insures that those dendritic cells which can interact successfully with naive T cells (i.e., those which are presenting the T cell's cognate antigen) will stick around long enough to activate lots of these T cells. So the interaction between the dendritic cell and a naive helper T cell is not just one way. These cells actually perform an activation "dance" in which they stimulate each other. The end result of this dance is that the dendritic cell becomes a more potent antigen presenting cell, and the Th cell is activated to express the high levels of CD40L required for helping activate B cells.

After activation is complete, the helper T cell and the antigen presenting cell part. The APC then goes on to activate other T cells, while the recently activated Th cells proliferate to build up their numbers. This proliferation is driven by growth factors such as IL-2. Naive T cells can produce some IL-2, but they don't have IL-2 receptors on their surface, so they can't respond to this cytokine. However, when Th cells are activated, growth factor receptors appear on their surfaces, and these cells begin to produce even larger amounts of IL-2. Consequently, newly activated helper T cells stimulate their own proliferation and double their numbers roughly every six hours. This coupling of activation to the upregulation of growth factor receptors is the essence of clonal selection: Those Th cells that are selected for activation (because their TCRs recognize an invader) upregulate their growth factor receptors, and proliferate to form a clone.

So the sequence of events during the activation of a helper T cell is: Adhesion molecules mediate weak binding between the Th and the APC while TCRs engage their cognate antigen presented by the APC. Receptor engagement strengthens the adhesion between the two cells, and upregulates CD40L expression on the Th cell. CD40L then binds to CD40 on the APC and stimulates expression of MHC and co-stimulatory molecules on the APC surface. The co-stimulation provided by the APC amplifies the "TCR engaged" signal, making activation more efficient. When activation is complete, the cells disengage, and the Th cell proliferates, driven by growth factors which bind to receptors that appear on the Th cell surface as a result of activation.

CYTOKINES SECRETED BY Th CELLS

When virgin helper T cells are first activated, the major cytokine they secrete is IL-2. Once Th cells have proliferated to build up a clone of identical cells, they may be re-stimulated by an APC, and begin to secrete other cytokines such as IFN-γ, IL-4, IL-5, IL-10, and TNF. Generally, a single Th cell doesn't secrete all these different cytokines. In fact, Th cells tend to secrete subsets of the possible cytokines. These subsets frequently are of two general types: a "Th1" subset that includes IL-2, IFN-γ, and TNF; and a "Th2" subset that includes interleukins 4, 5, and 10.

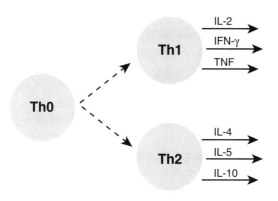

You shouldn't take this to mean, however, that there are only two subsets of cytokines that can be secreted by Th cells. In fact, immunologists initially had a hard time finding helper cells that secreted exactly the Th1 or Th2 cytokine subsets in humans. Clearly, there are Th cells which secrete mixtures of cytokines that <u>don't</u> conform to the Th1/Th2 paradigm, but the concept of Th1 and Th2 subsets turns out to be quite useful in trying to make sense of the mixture of cytokines (the cytokine "profile") that Th cells produce.

Why do you think it makes sense for different Th cells to secrete different subsets of the possible cytokines? Let me review the functions of the cytokines that make up the Th1 and Th2 subsets, and I think you'll soon understand what Mother Nature is up to.

The "classical" Th1 cytokines are IFN-γ, IL-2, and TNF. IFN-γ is a cytokine that primes macrophages and influences B cells during class switching to produce IgG3 antibodies that are good at opsonizing viruses and bacteria and at fixing complement. TNF activates primed macrophages and natural killer cells, and IL-2 is a growth factor that stimulates CTLs and NK cells to proliferate. So the Th1 cytokines are the perfect package to help defend against a viral or bacterial attack in the blood and tissues because Th1 cytokines instruct the innate and adaptive systems to produce cells and antibodies that are especially effective against these invaders.

Next let's look at the Th2 profile of cytokines. IL-4 is a growth factor for B cells that can also influence B

cells to class switch to produce IgE antibodies. IL-5 is a cytokine that can encourage B cells to produce IgA antibodies. So the Th2 cytokine profile is just the ticket if you need to make lots of antibodies to defend against a parasitic (IgE) or mucosal (IgA) infection.

What's happening here is that, as the "quarterback" of the immune system team, the helper T cell, "calls the plays" by secreting cytokines which direct the immune response. By secreting the appropriate set of cytokines, Th cells can help orchestrate an immune response that is appropriate for a given invader – so that the punishment fits the crime.

Now there is one very important point here that I want to make sure you understand. When we talk about influencing the immune response toward a Th1 or Th2 cytokine profile, we are talking about something very local. Clearly, you wouldn't want every Th cell in your body to be of the Th1 type, because then you'd have no way to defend against a respiratory infection. Conversely, you wouldn't want to have only Th2 cells, because the IgA or IgE antibodies made in response to the Th2 cytokines would be useless if you get a bacterial infection in your big toe. In fact, it is the local nature of cytokine signaling which gives the immune system the flexibility to simultaneously mount defenses against many different invaders that threaten different parts of the body.

THE DENDRITIC CELL AS "COACH" OF THE IMMUNE SYSTEM TEAM

Okay, so helper T cells use cytokines to direct the immune response. But how do these quarterback cells know which cytokines are appropriate for a given situation? To make an informed decision on which cytokines to make, at least two pieces of information are required. First, it's necessary to know what type of invader the immune system is dealing with. Is it a virus, a bacterium, or a parasite? Second, it's essential to determine where in the body the invaders are located. Are they in the respiratory tract, the digestive tract, or the big toe? Virgin helper T cells don't have direct access to either type of information. After all, they are busy circulating through the blood and lymph trying to find their cognate antigens. What's needed is an "observer" who has actually been at the battle site, who has collected the pertinent information, and who can pass it along to the helper T cell. And which of the immune system cells could qualify as such an observer? The dendritic antigen presenting cell, of course!

Just as the coach of a football team collects information on the opposing team and formulates a game plan, so the dendritic cell, acting as "coach" of the immune system team, collects information on the invasion and decides how the immune system should react. That's why dendritic cells are so important. They don't just turn helper T cells and killer T cells on. They actually function as the "brains" of the immune system, processing all the inputs pertaining to the invasion, and producing a plan of action.

What are the inputs that dendritic cells integrate to produce the game plan? Immunologists have now identified two different types of "intelligence" that is collected by dendritic cells out at the battle scene. The first type of input is received through receptors on the surfaces of dendritic cells which recognize, either directly or indirectly, molecular "patterns" that are characteristic of broad classes of invaders. So far the most carefully studied of these are the "Toll-like" receptors. For example, Toll-like receptor 4 (TLR4) senses the presence of LPS, the molecules we have already talked about which are components of the coats of Gram-negative bacteria. In addition, TLR4 can detect proteins made by certain viruses. TLR2 also can recognize certain forms of LPS, but this receptor specializes in identifying proteins that are "signatures" of Gram-positive bacteria. TLR3 recognizes the double-stranded RNA produced during many viral infections. And TLR9 recognizes the unmethylated DNA dinucleotide, CpG, that is characteristic of bacterial DNA. Dendritic cells also have receptors that detect "heat shock proteins" – proteins which cells release when they are stressed or dying. It is thought that by sensing the presence of these heat shock proteins, dendritic cells can be alerted that cells in their neighborhood are being killed by viruses.

Although it is certain that many more receptors of this type will be discovered, the emerging picture is that the surfaces of dendritic cells (and macrophages) are studded with receptors that are "tuned" to recognize various structural features of common microbial invaders. Some invaders can trigger several different receptors, so there is overlap and redundancy built into this recognition system. Although still somewhat speculative, it is likely that dendritic cells standing guard in different parts of the body express different combinations of these pattern receptors.

Because different pathogens elicit the production of different cytokines during an infection, dendritic cells also can learn a lot about the invader by sensing the cytokine environment. In addition, different areas of the body (e.g., skin vs. mucosa) produce characteristic mixtures of cytokines in response to invaders, and this information helps the dendritic cell identify the area of the body that is under attack. Consequently, the second type of input that dendritic cells "listen to" when formulating their game plans is collected by surface receptors that respond to various cytokines.

So dendritic cells out on the front lines receive input about the invader through pattern recognition receptors and cytokine receptors. It is then up to the dendritic cell to "decode" these inputs and decide what types of weapons need to be mobilized and where they need to be sent. But how is the game plan that is synthesized by the dendritic cell conveyed to the Th cell – the cell that will direct the action? Again, a detailed answer to this question is not available, but a picture is emerging. Although B7 is the best-studied co-stimulatory molecule expressed by activated dendritic cells, other co-stimulatory molecules have been identified, and more such molecules will certainly be discovered. In addition to surface molecules like B7, cytokines produced by activated dendritic cells also can have co-stimulatory activity. The bottom line is that when an activated dendritic cell reaches a lymph node, it expresses a number of different co-stimulatory molecules. And the particular collection of co-stimulatory molecules that a dendritic cell "offers" to a naive Th cell in the lymph node will depend on the "scouting report" the dendritic cell received at the battle scene. It is this collection of co-stimulatory signals which conveys the "game plan" to the virgin helper T cell.

To summarize, dendritic cells are stationed beneath all exposed surfaces, where they wait for information on the identities of various invaders that may breach the barrier defenses. This information is collected by receptors on the dendritic cell surfaces – receptors which recognize either molecular patterns that are characteristic of classes of invaders, or cytokines produced by other cells in response to the invasion. The dendritic cell then integrates all this information, travels to a nearby lymph node, and by expressing certain combinations of co-stimulatory molecules, delivers a game plan to helper T cells that informs them what weapons to mobilize and where to deliver these weapons.

It is important to remember that dendritic cells are members of the innate system team. Thus, the innate immune system not only informs the adaptive system when there is danger, but it also "coaches" the adaptive system so that the appropriate weapons are sent to the right places.

A HELPER T CELL'S LIFE AFTER ACTIVATION

Once a naive helper T cell has been activated by a dendritic cell, it proliferates rapidly for a few days. Members of this clone of activated Th cells may then be re-stimulated by other dendritic cells in the lymph node and proliferate some more. Of course, if being simulated and proliferating were all Th cells did, they would be pretty useless. So eventually (usually in less than a week) these Th cells get enough of this fun, and "mature" into what immunologists call "effector" cells – cells that can actually do something. Let me explain.

Effector helper T cells have two main duties. First, they can remain in the blood and lymphatic circulation and travel from node to node, providing help for B cells or for cytotoxic T cells. The other duty of an effector helper T cell is to exit blood vessels at sites where there is a battle going on to provide help for the "soldiers" of the innate and adaptive immune systems. The initial cytokine profile that effector Th cells express is determined mainly by the co-stimulation they receive during the activation phase. For example, based on this co-stimulation, helper T cells may "decide" to secrete Th1 or Th2 subsets of cytokines. Other helper T cells (the so-called "Th0" cells) may remain unbiased, being able to produce a wide range of cytokines.

Once the effector cells reach the battle scene, however, their commitment to a certain cytokine profile can either be changed or reinforced. For instance, out at the front, activated macrophages responding to a bacterial or viral invasion will secrete IL-12. This is the major cytokine that influences Th cells to secrete the Th1 profile of cytokines. So when newly activated Th cells exit the blood in an environment rich in IL-12, uncommitted (Th0) helper cells "realize" what type of battle is being fought, and are influenced to produce the Th1 cytokines (IFN-γ, IL-2, and TNF) that are needed to defend against bacteria or viruses. In addition, the high concentration of IL-12 at the battle site will strengthen the commitment of helper cells that had already decided to secrete a Th1 cytokine profile.

In contrast, if Th cells exit the blood at a site where a parasitic invasion is being dealt with, they will find themselves in an environment rich in IL-4. This cytokine encourages uncommitted helper T cells to produce Th2 cytokines (IL-4, IL-5, and IL-10), which are perfect for helping battle a parasitic infection. In addition, the high concentration of IL-4 reinforces the decision of Th cells that are already committed to a Th2 cytokine profile to continue in this direction.

Committed Th cells can also influence the cytokine profile produced by other Th cells in the neighborhood. In this sense, helper T cells are like "evangelists" who try to "convert" other Th cells to their "religion." For example, Th1 cells secrete IFN-γ, which together with danger signals like the bacterial molecule LPS, helps activate macrophages. These activated macrophages then secrete IL-12, which influences uncommitted (Th0) helper T cells to become Th1 cells.

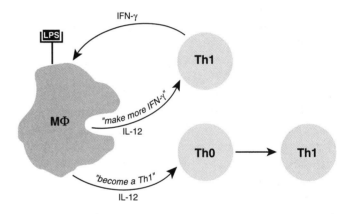

Th2 cells also are evangelists, because these cells secrete IL-4, which influences Th0 cells to produce the Th2 profile of cytokines. So in both cases, cytokines secreted by committed Th cells either directly or indirectly recruit other, uncommitted Th cells to secrete the same mixture of cytokines.

Once a Th cell has made a choice, it begins to produce its own growth factor: Th1 cells secrete IL-2, which is a growth factor that drives Th1 cell proliferation; and Th2 cells secrete their favorite growth factor, IL-4, that causes them to proliferate. So not only do the cytokines secreted by each subset encourage new Th cells to fall into step, but these cytokines also cause the selected Th cells to proliferate to build up their numbers.

Finally, there is also <u>negative</u> feedback at work. IFN-γ made by Th1 cells actually decreases the rate of proliferation of Th2 cells, so that fewer Th2 cells will be produced.

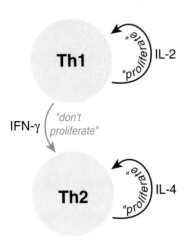

On the other side of the picture, one of the Th2 cytokines, IL-10, acts to decrease the rate of proliferation of Th1 cells.

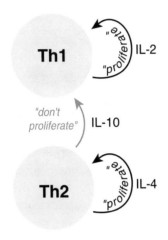

The bottom line here is that once a Th cytokine profile has been established, positive and negative feedback tend to "lock in" this particular profile. This clever strategy of beginning with a combination of committed and uncommitted helper T cells that can subsequently become strongly biased toward the production of a certain subset of cytokines gives the system the flexibility to respond locally to many different microbes that may invade more or less simultaneously. Once Th cells have reached the battle scene, the combination of positive and negative feedback focuses the <u>local</u> immune response on the invader at hand by ensuring that most of the helper T cells there end up "on the same page."

DELAYED TYPE HYPERSENSITIVITY

There is an example of "signal calling" by Th cells that I think you'll find interesting. It's termed "delayed type hypersensitivity" (DTH), and it was first observed by Robert Koch when he was studying tuberculosis back in the latter part of the nineteenth century. Koch purified a protein, tuberculin, from the bacterium that causes tuberculosis, and used this protein to devise his famous "tuberculin skin test." If you've had this test, you'll recall that a nurse injected something under your skin, and told you to check that area in a few days. If the spot where you were injected became red and swollen, you were instructed to come back in to see the doctor. Here's what that's all about.

The "something" you were injected with was Koch's tuberculin protein. When dendritic cells beneath your skin (the so-called "Langerhans" cells) take up tuberculin, they cut it up into pieces, and use class II MHC molecules to display fragments of this protein. Dendritic cells in the tissues express enough MHC and B7 molecules to re-stimulate memory (experienced) T cells, but not enough of these molecules to activate naive T cells. If you have active TB or have been infected with it in the past, your immune system will include memory, Th1-type helper T cells. These cells can recognize the tuberculin fragments presented by the dendritic cells stationed beneath the skin and be re-activated. Now the fun begins, because these Th cells begin to secrete IFN-γ and TNF – Th1-type cytokines that activate resident tissue macrophages near the site of injection, and help recruit neutrophils and additional macrophages to the area. The result is a local inflammatory reaction with the redness and swelling: the signal that your TB test is positive. Of course, the reason you have to wait several days for the test to "develop" is that memory helper T cells must be re-activated, proliferate, and produce those all-important cytokines that orchestrate the inflammatory reaction.

On the other hand, if you have never been exposed to the tuberculosis bacterium, you will have no memory helper T cells to re-activate. Without the cytokines supplied by activated Th cells, there will be no inflammatory reaction to the tuberculin protein, and your skin test will be scored as negative.

What is interesting here is that delayed type hypersensitivity is both specific and non-specific. The specificity comes from Th cells that direct the immune response after recognizing the tuberculin peptide presented by dendritic cells. The non-specific part of the reaction includes neutrophils and macrophages that are recruited and activated by cytokines secreted by the Th cells. This is yet another example of the cooperation that goes on between adaptive and innate immune systems.

Now, you may be wondering why the tuberculin used for the test doesn't activate naive T cells, so that the next time you are tested, you would get a positive reaction. The reason is that the tuberculin protein does not by itself cause an inflammatory reaction (i.e., a battle situation), and you remember that dendritic cells only carry antigen to a lymph node if a battle is on. So if a protein is injected under your skin and does not cause inflammation (i.e., is ignored by the innate system) dendritic cells won't travel to lymph nodes to activate the adaptive immune response. This illustrates again how important the innate immune system is for <u>initiating</u> an immune response: If your innate system does not recognize an invader as dangerous and put up a fight, your adaptive system usually will just ignore the invasion.

HOW KILLER T CELLS ARE ACTIVATED

So far our discussion has focused on helper T cells – how they are activated and what they do. Now we need to look more closely at killer T cells, because the way they are activated in lymph nodes is different from the way Th cells are activated – and, of course, what CTLs do once they are activated is very different from what Th cells do.

Although the steps involved in activating helper T cells are now fairly well understood, the activation of killer T cells still is a bit mysterious. One of the problems is that, in most cases, activation of a virgin CTL requires not only that it recognize its cognate antigen presented by class I MHC molecules on a dendritic cell, but that it receive help from a helper T cell as well. One way to solve this problem would be for the dendritic cell, the Th cell, and the CTL to engage in a *ménage à trois*. However, just as a successful *ménage à trois* is rare in real life, so too the probability that a helper T cell and a killer T cell will <u>simultaneously</u> find a dendritic cell that is presenting their cognate antigen is extremely small.

Recently, a new hypothesis has been forwarded to deal with the improbability of a three-cell interaction. According to this proposal, a dendritic cell can activate a helper T cell and a CTL <u>sequentially</u>. The idea is that during the "dance" which results in the activation of the Th cell, the dendritic cell somehow becomes "licensed" to subsequently activate killer T cells – those CTLs that drop by later and which recognize their cognate antigens displayed by the licensed dendritic cell.

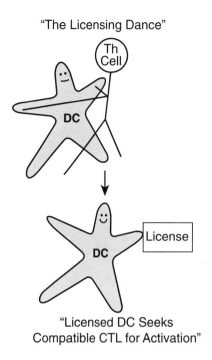

"The Licensing Dance"

"Licensed DC Seeks
Compatible CTL for Activation"

So far, the mechanisms involved in licensing remain unknown. As we discussed earlier, the dance between a Th cell and a dendritic cell can increase the level of expression of class I MHC and co-stimulatory molecules on the surface of the dendritic cell, and can cause the dendritic cell to secrete cytokines. So it may be that the dendritic cell leaves the dance floor with more of the goodies required to activate a naive killer T cell – but this is just a guess.

THE LIFE OF A CTL AFTER ACTIVATION

Once a CTL has been activated, it proliferates rapidly to build up its numbers. Then, it leaves the lymph node, enters the blood, and searches for the area of the body where the invaders it can kill are located. When it finds the battle site, it exits the blood, and begins to hack away at infected cells. Most killing by CTLs requires contact between the CTL and its target cell, and CTLs have several weapons they can use during this "hand-to-hand" combat. One involves the production of the protein, perforin. Perforin is a close relative of the C9 complement protein that is part of the membrane attack complex, and perforin can bind to cellular membranes and make holes in them. The latest thinking is that when a CTL uses perforin to kill, its TCRs first identify the target. Then adhesion molecules on the CTL hold the target cell close while the killer cell delivers a mixture of perforin and an enzyme called granzyme B onto the surface of the target cell. The target cell's reaction is to enclose the granzyme and the perforin in a pouch (vesicle) made from the target cell's membrane and to take them inside.

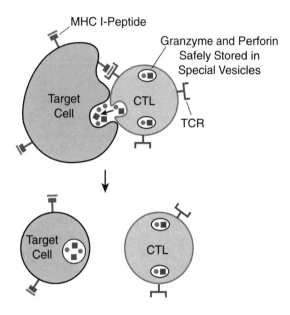

Once inside the target cell, the perforin molecules make holes in the vesicle, allowing the granzyme B to escape into the cytoplasm of the cell. There granzyme B triggers an enzymatic chain reaction that causes the cell to commit suicide by apoptosis. This kind of "assisted suicide" usually involves the self-destruction of the target cell's DNA by its own enzymes.

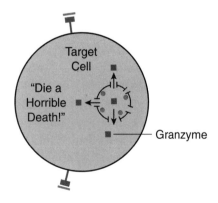

CTLs also can kill by using a protein on their surfaces called Fas ligand (FasL) that can bind to (ligate) the Fas protein on the surface of a target cell. When this happens, a suicide program is set in motion within the target cell, and again, the cell dies by apoptosis.

Actually, there are two different ways that a cell can die: by necrosis or by apoptosis. Although the end result is the same (a dead cell), what happens when cells die by necrosis or apoptosis is quite different. Cells usually die of necrosis either as the result of a wound (e.g., a cut or a burn) or when they are destroyed by an attacking virus or bacterium. During necrosis, enzymes and chemicals that normally are safely contained within a living cell are released into the surrounding tissues where they can do real damage. In contrast, death by apoptosis is much cleaner. As a cell dies by apoptosis, its contents are enclosed in vesicles made from the walls of the dying cell. These vesicles are then eaten and destroyed by nearby macrophages as part of their garbage collecting duty. Consequently, during apoptosis, the contents of the target cell don't get out into the tissues to cause damage. So by "choosing" to kill their targets by inducing apoptosis rather than necrosis, CTLs can rid the body of virus-infected cells without causing the collateral tissue damage that would result from necrotic cell death.

There is another reason why triggering cells to die by apoptosis is an especially effective way for killer T cells to destroy virus-infected cells. When virus-infected cells die by apoptosis, the DNA of unassembled viruses is destroyed along with the target cell's DNA. In addition, viruses that have already been assembled inside the infected target cell are enclosed in apoptotic vesicles and are disposed of by macrophages. It is this ability to kill infected cells by inducing apoptosis that makes killer T cells such potent antiviral weapons.

Although a single CTL is capable of killing many target cells sequentially, during a virus attack thousands of cells may be infected. So to amplify their killing power, CTLs can proliferate once they reach the battle scene. Most CTLs depend on an external supply of IL-2 to proliferate – and Th1 cells are the major suppliers of this cytokine. Consequently, when many CTLs are needed (e.g., during a viral infection), helper T cells that secrete a Th1 cytokine profile can supply the IL-2 required for killer T cells to proliferate. In this way, helper T cells "call the plays," and control the strength of a killer T cell response.

MEMORY T CELLS

After they have been activated and have done their thing, most T cells are programmed to die by apoptosis. Immunologists call this activation induced cell death (ACID). This makes perfect sense, because we don't want our immune systems cluttered up with activated helper and killer T cells that can only defend against old invaders. ACID makes "room" for new T cells that can be activated in response to the next microbes that try to do us in.

On the other hand, it would be nice to have some of the old guys stick around, just in case we are attacked by the same invader again. Fortunately, the immune system has provided for this possibility by setting aside some of the T cells that are activated each time we are attacked as "memory cells." These cells are "wired" so that activation signals are very efficiently transmitted from the cell surface to the nucleus. Consequently, they can fire up quickly to protect us if their TCRs are engaged again by the invader they recognize.

So far, there is a great deal of mystery surrounding how activated T cells are "picked" to become memory cells. Some immunologists favor the idea that memory T cells are the ones that were only partially activated (whatever that means) during the first attack, whereas other immunologists prefer the hypothesis that memory T cells are selected (how, they aren't sure) from the pool of fully activated T cells. It is also not completely clear how these "survivors" are kept alive, once they become memory cells. The current view is that in response to cytokines, memory T cells proliferate slowly to maintain their numbers – even after their cognate antigens have been eliminated from the body. So although it is clear that memory T cells do provide long-term protection against future attacks, there is still a lot to be discovered about how these memory cells are chosen and maintained.

EPILOGUE

As we come to the end of this lecture, you should now be familiar with all of the major players of the innate and adaptive immune systems. As I'm sure you now understand, these players form a "network" in which they work together to defend us from disease. For this network to function, however, the movements of the various players must be carefully choreographed to enhance cooperation between players, and to make sure that the appropriate weapons are delivered to the locations within the body where they are needed. How all this is accomplished is the subject of our next lecture.

SUMMARY FIGURE

Here is our final summary figure, showing both the innate and adaptive systems – and the network they form. Can you identify all the players, and do you understand how they interact with each other?

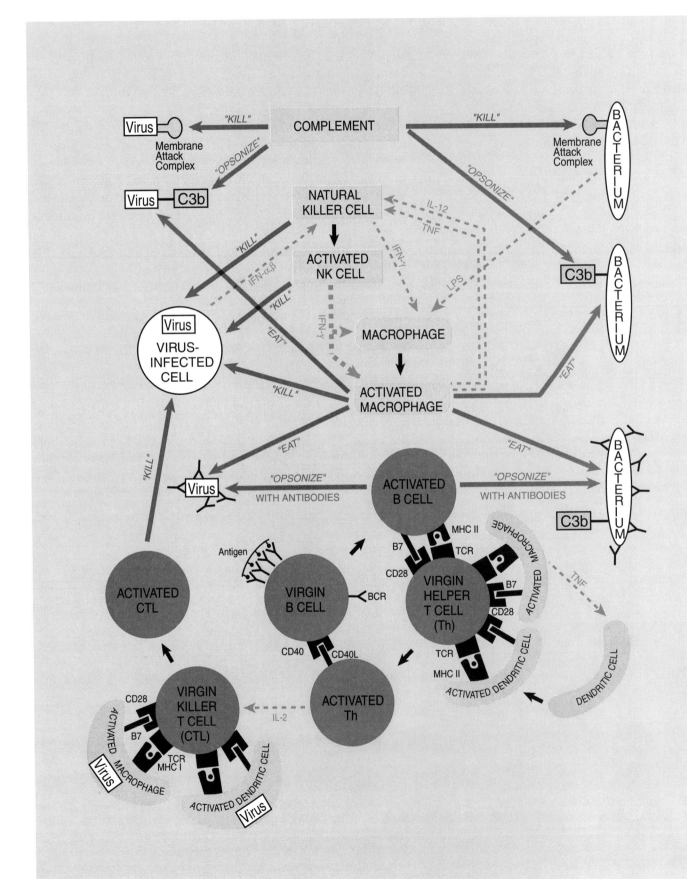

THOUGHT QUESTIONS

1. Essentially all players on the innate and adaptive immune system teams must be activated before they can "get in the game." Trace the steps in the "activation cascade" that begins when an LPS-carrying, Gram-negative bacterium enters a wound, and that ends when antibodies are produced that can recognize the bacterium.

2. What happens when dendritic cells and helper T cells "dance"?

3. How does a helper T cell know which cytokine profile to produce?

4. How does a helper T cell "call the plays" for B cells?

5. How does a helper T cell "call the plays" for killer T cells?

6. Why is it that some people seem to have a "good" immune system (i.e., they never get sick), whereas others seem to catch every bug that comes along? Asked another way: Which components of the immune system can differ between individuals?

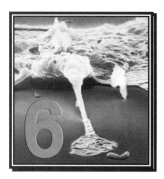

LYMPHOID ORGANS AND LYMPHOCYTE TRAFFICKING

REVIEW

I'm sure you noticed during the last lecture that there are many similarities between T cells and B cells. As a way of reviewing, let's recall some of the ways that T and B cells are similar – and different.

BCRs and TCRs both have "recognition" proteins that extend outside the cell, and which are incredibly diverse because they are made by a strategy of mixing and matching gene segments. For the BCR, these are the light and heavy chains that make up the antibody molecule. For the TCR, the molecules that recognize antigen are the α and β or γ and δ proteins. TCRs and BCRs have cytoplasmic tails that are too short to signal recognition, so additional molecules are required for this purpose. For the BCR, these signaling proteins are called Igα and Igβ, while for the TCR, signaling involves a complex of proteins called CD3.

For B and T cells to be activated, their receptors must be clustered by antigen, because this crosslinking brings together many of their signaling molecules in a small region of the cell. When the density of signaling molecules is great enough, an enzymatic chain reaction is set off that conveys the "receptor engaged" signal to the cell's nucleus. There, in the "brain center" of the cell, genes involved in activation are turned off or on as a result of this signal. Although crosslinking of receptors is essential for activation, it is not enough. Naive B and T cells also require co-stimulatory signals that are not antigen specific. For B cell activation, a helper T cell can provide co-stimulation through surface proteins called CD40L that plug into CD40 proteins on the B cell surface. For T cells, one form of co-stimulation involves B7 proteins on an antigen presenting cell that engage CD28 proteins on the surface of the T cell.

In addition to recognition and signaling molecules, BCRs and TCRs also associate with co-receptor molecules that serve to amplify the signal that the receptors send. For B cells, this co-receptor is one which recognizes antigen that has been opsonized by complement. If the BCR recognizes an antigen, and if that antigen is also "decorated" with complement protein fragments, the antigen serves as a "clamp" that brings the BCR and the complement receptor together on the surface of the B cell, greatly amplifying the "receptor engaged" signal. As a consequence, B cells are much more easily activated (many fewer BCRs must be crosslinked) by antigen that has been opsonized by complement.

T cells also have co-receptors: Th cells express CD4 molecules on their surfaces, and CTLs express CD8 molecules. When a TCR binds to antigen presented by MHC proteins, the co-receptor molecule on the T cell surface also binds to the MHC molecule. This serves to amplify the signal that is sent by the TCR to the nucleus, so that the T cell is more easily activated (fewer TCRs must be crosslinked). Of course, these co-receptors only work with the "right" MHC types: class I for CTLs with CD8 co-receptors and class II for Th cells with CD4 co-receptors.

So co-receptors are really "focus" molecules. The B cell co-receptor helps B cells focus on antigens that have already been identified by the complement system as dangerous (those that have been opsonized). The CD4 co-receptor focuses the attention of Th cells on antigens displayed by class II MHC molecules, and the CD8 co-receptor focuses CTLs on antigens displayed by class I MHC molecules.

When B and T cells are activated, growth factor receptors appear on their surfaces. This allows them to proliferate in response to the appropriate growth factors, and to form a clone of cells that has the same antigen specificity. B and Th cells are also similar in that when they are re-stimulated, they get a chance to change the molecules they secrete. B cells can undergo class switching to produce IgG, IgA, or IgE antibodies in place of the default antibody class, IgM. Helper T cells can secrete a whole list of cytokines in addition to, or instead of, the default cytokine IL-2. For B cells, the change in antibody class is influenced by cytokines present in the local environment when the decision to change classes is made. For helper T cells, the decision to produce certain cytokines is determined both by the type of co-stimulation the Th cell receives and by the cytokine milieu.

There are also important differences between B cells and T cells. The BCR recognizes antigen in its "natural" state – that is, antigen that has not been chopped up and bound to MHC molecules. This antigen can be a protein or almost any other organic molecule (e.g., a carbohydrate or a fat). In contrast, the αβ receptors on a T cell only recognize fragments of proteins that are presented by MHC molecules. So the BCR has much greater variety in the type of antigen it can recognize. However, because the TCR looks at small fragments of proteins, it can recognize targets that are hidden from view of the BCR in an intact and tightly folded protein.

Of course, B and T cells have different functions. B cells secrete antibodies – a non-membrane-anchored form of the BCR. In contrast, the TCR stays firmly anchored on the surface of the T cell. Experienced B cells can function as antigen presenting cells, but T cells cannot. CTLs are killers, but B cells do not kill. Finally, Th cells are major cytokine producers, whereas B cells usually produce cytokines only in small amounts.

During an infection, the parts of the rearranged heavy and light chain genes that specify the antigen binding region of the B cell receptor can undergo somatic hypermutation and selection. As a result, the average affinity of the collection of BCRs increases. So in a sense, B cells can "draw from the deck" to try to get a better hand. In contrast, the TCR does not hypermutate, so T cells must be satisfied with the cards they are dealt. B cells are produced more or less continuously throughout the lifetime of a human, but the production of virgin T cells decreases as a person ages. The reason is that the organ in which T cells mature, the thymus, steadily decreases in activity after puberty, so fewer and fewer freshly minted T cells roll off the thymic assembly line as we get older. That's one reason why some viral diseases such as mumps, which are just a nuisance to a kid, can be deadly serious to an older person.

Certainly one of the most elegant features of the immune system is the way Mother Nature arranges to "let the punishment fit the crime." Dendritic antigen presenting cells observe the battle first hand, and the intelligence they gather there is complete enough to allow them to formulate a "game plan." Once activated, dendritic cells travel to nearby lymph nodes, where they activate T cells. During this process, the game plan is conveyed to T cells in the form of co-stimulatory molecules (including cytokines) that are expressed by the dendritic cells. This information instructs helper T cells which cytokines to make to defend against a particular invader, and informs both Th cells and CTLs where in the body they should travel to join in the fight. In a sense, the dendritic cell functions as the "coach" of the immune system team, while the Th cell performs the duties of "quarterback" by calling the plays designed by the coach. It is important to note that the cell that functions as coach is actually part of the innate immune system. So the innate system determines not only when the adaptive system should be activated in response to danger, but also instructs the adaptive system on which weapons to deploy and where to send them.

SECONDARY LYMPHOID ORGANS AND LYMPHOCYTE TRAFFICKING

Up to this point, we've discussed the various elements of innate and adaptive immunity, and how they interact to make an integrated defense "system." However, to really understand how the immune system works, one must have a clear picture of where in the body all these interactions take place. So in this lecture, we're going to focus on the "geography" of the immune system.

The immune system's defense against an invader

actually has three phases: recognition of danger, production of weapons appropriate for the invader, and transport of these weapons to the site of attack. The recognition phase of the adaptive immune response takes place in the so-called "secondary lymphoid organs." These include the lymph nodes, the spleen, and the mucosal-associated lymphoid tissue (called the MALT for short). You may be wondering: If these are the secondary lymphoid organs, what are the primary ones? The primary lymphoid organs are the bone marrow, where B and T cells are born, and the thymus, where T cells receive their early training.

LYMPHOID FOLLICLES

All secondary lymphoid organs have one anatomical feature in common: They all contain lymphoid follicles. These follicles are critical for the functioning of the adaptive immune system, so we need to spend a little time getting familiar with them. Lymphoid follicles start life as "primary" lymphoid follicles: loose networks of follicular dendritic cells (FDCs) embedded in regions of the secondary lymphoid organs that are rich in B cells. So lymphoid follicles are really islands of follicular dendritic cells within a sea of B cells.

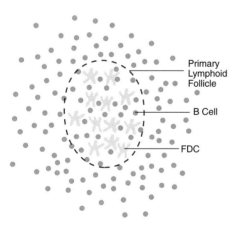

Although FDCs have the classic "starfish" dendritic shape, they are very different from the antigen presenting dendritic cells (DCs) of the skin and mucosa that we have talked about before. Those dendritic cells are white blood cells that are produced in the bone marrow, and which then migrate to their sentinel posi-

tions in the tissues. In contrast, follicular dendritic cells are regular old cells (like skin cells or liver cells) that take up their final positions in the secondary lymphoid organs as the embryo develops. In fact, follicular dendritic cells are already in place during the second trimester of gestation. Not only are the origins of follicular dendritic cells and antigen presenting dendritic cells quite different, these two types of starfish-shaped cells have very different functions. Whereas the role of dendritic APCs is to present antigen to T cells via MHC molecules, the function of follicular dendritic cells is to display antigen to B cells. Here's how this works.

Early in an infection, complement proteins bind to invaders, and some of this complement-opsonized antigen will be delivered by the lymph or blood to the secondary lymphoid organs. Follicular dendritic cells that reside in these organs have receptors on their surfaces that bind to complement fragments, and as a result, follicular dendritic cells pick up and retain the opsonized antigen. In this way, follicular dendritic cells become "decorated" with antigens that are derived from the battle that is being waged out in the tissues. Later during the battle, when antibodies have been produced, invaders opsonized by antibodies also can be captured by FDCs, because these cells have receptors that can bind to the constant regions of antibody molecules. By capturing large numbers of antigens and by holding them close together, FDCs display antigens in a way that can crosslink B cell receptors.

So follicular dendritic cells capture opsonized antigens and "advertise" these antigens to B cells in a configuration that can help activate them. Those B cells whose receptors are crosslinked by their cognate antigens hanging from these follicular dendritic "trees" are retained for a while in the lymphoid follicle, where they proliferate to build up their numbers. Once this happens, the "follicle" begins to grow and to become the center of B cell development. Such an active lymphoid follicle is called a "secondary" lymphoid follicle or a "germinal center." The role of complement-opsonized antigen in triggering the development of a germinal center cannot be overemphasized: Lymphoid follicles in humans who have a defective complement system never progress past the primary stage. Thus, we see again that for the adaptive immune system to respond, the innate system must first react to impending danger.

As B cells proliferate in germinal centers, they become very "fragile." Unless they receive the proper "rescue" signals, they will commit suicide (die by apoptosis). Fortunately, helper T cells that have been activated in the T cell areas of the secondary lymphoid organs migrate to the lymphoid follicle to rescue these B cells. Activated Th cells express high levels of CD40L proteins that can plug into CD40 proteins on the surface of the B cell. When a B cell whose receptors are crosslinked by antigen receives this co-stimulatory signal, it is temporarily rescued from apoptotic death, and continues to proliferate.

The rate at which B cells multiply in a germinal center is truly amazing – the number of B cells can double every six hours! These proliferating B cells push aside other B cells that have not been activated, and establish a region of the germinal center that is called the "dark zone" – because it contains so many proliferating B cells that it looks dark under the microscope.

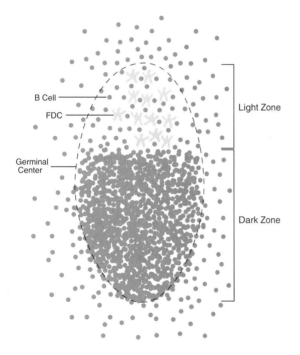

After this period of proliferation, some of the B cells "choose" to become plasma B cells and leave the germinal center. Others undergo somatic hypermutation. After each round of mutation, the affinity of the mutated BCR is tested. Those B cells whose mutated BCRs do not have a high enough affinity for antigen will die by apoptosis, and will be eaten by macrophages in the germinal center. In contrast, B cells are rescued from apoptosis if their receptors have a high enough affinity to be efficiently crosslinked by antigen on FDCs, and if they also receive co-stimulation from activated Th cells

that are present in the light zone of the germinal center. The current picture is that B cells "cycle" between periods of proliferation in the dark zone and periods of testing in the light zone. Sometime during all this action, B cells can also switch the class of antibody they produce. This process is believed to take place in the light zone of the germinal center with the aid of activated Th cells.

In summary, lymphoid follicles are specialized regions of secondary lymphoid organs in which B cells percolate through a lattice of follicular dendritic cells that have captured opsonized antigen on their surfaces. B cells that encounter their cognate antigen and receive T cell help are rescued from death. These "saved" B cells proliferate and can undergo somatic hypermutation and class switching. Clearly, lymphoid follicles are extremely important for B cell development. That's why all secondary lymphoid organs have them.

HIGH ENDOTHELIAL VENULES

A second anatomical feature common to all secondary lymphoid organs except the spleen is the "high endothelial venule" (HEV). The reason HEVs are so important is that they are the "doorways" through which B and T cells enter these secondary lymphoid organs from the blood. Most endothelial cells that line the inside of blood vessels resemble overlapping shingles that are tightly "glued" to the cells adjacent to them to prevent the loss of blood cells into the tissues. In contrast, the blood vessels that collect blood from the capillary beds (the post-capillary venules) in most secondary lymphoid organs are lined with special endothelial cells that are shaped more like a column than like a shingle.

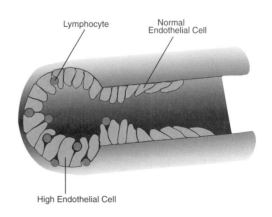

These tall cells are the high endothelial cells. So a high endothelial venule is a special region in a blood vessel (venule) where there are high endothelial cells. Instead of being glued together, high endothelial cells are "spot welded." As a result, there is enough space between the cells of the HEV for lymphocytes to wriggle through. Actually, "wriggle" may not be quite the right term, because lymphocytes exit the blood very efficiently at these high endothelial venules: About 10,000 lymphocytes exit the blood and enter an average lymph node each second by passing between high endothelial cells!

A TOUR OF THE SECONDARY LYMPHOID ORGANS

Now that you are familiar with lymphoid follicles and high endothelial venules, we are ready to take a tour of some of the secondary lymphoid organs. On our tour today, we will visit a lymph node, a Peyer's patch (an example of the MALT), and the spleen. As we explore these organs, you will want to pay special attention to the "plumbing." How an organ is plumbed gives important clues about how it functions.

LYMPH NODES

The lymph node is a plumber's dream. This organ has incoming lymphatics, which bring lymph into the node, and outgoing lymphatics through which lymph exits the node. In addition, there are small arteries (arterioles) that carry the blood that nourishes the cells of the lymph node, and veins through which this blood leaves the node. If you look carefully at this figure, you can also see the high endothelial venules.

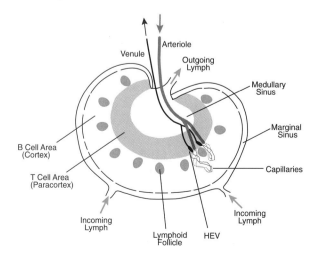

With this plumbing in mind, can you see how B and T cells enter the lymph node? That's right, they can enter via the blood by pushing their way between the cells of the high endothelial venules. There is also another way lymphocytes can enter the lymph node. Do you see it? Of course – through the lymph. After all, lymph nodes are "dating bars," positioned along the route the lymph takes on its way to be reunited with the blood. And lymphocytes actively engage in "bar hopping," being carried from node to node by the lymph. Although lymphocytes have two ways to gain entry to a lymph node, they only exit via the lymph – those high endothelial venules won't let them back into the blood.

Since lymph nodes are places where lymphocytes find their cognate antigens, we also need to discuss how antigens enter a node. When dendritic cells stationed out in the tissues are stimulated by battle cytokines, they leave the tissues via the lymph, and carry antigens they have acquired at the battle scene into the secondary lymphoid organs. So this is one way antigen can enter a lymph node: as "cargo" aboard APCs. In addition, antigen that has been opsonized by complement or antibodies can be carried by the lymph into the node. There the opsonized antigen can be captured by follicular dendritic cells for display to B cells. When lymph enters the node, it percolates through holes in the marginal sinus (sinus is a fancy word for cavity), through the cortex and paracortex, and finally into the medullary sinus where it is collected so it can exit the node via the outgoing lymphatic vessels.

The walls of the marginal sinus are lined with macrophages that are tasked with cleaning up the lymph, so one of the functions of a lymph node is as a "lymph filter." Incidentally, when surgeons remove a cancer from some organ in the body, they generally inspect the lymph nodes that drain the lymph from that organ. If they find cancer cells in the draining lymph nodes, it is an indication that the cancer has begun to metastasize to other parts of the body, the first stop being the nearby lymph nodes.

The high endothelial venules are located in the paracortex, so lymphocytes pass through this region of the node when they arrive from the blood. In fact, T cells tend to accumulate in the paracortex, being retained there by adhesion molecules. This accumulation of T cells makes good sense, because dendritic cells are also found in the paracortex – and of course, one object of this game is to get T cells together with these antigen presenting cells.

As a helper T cell passes through the paracortex of the lymph node, there is a chance it will encounter a dendritic cell that is presenting its cognate antigen. If so, the Th cell will be activated and will begin to proliferate. This proliferation phase lasts a few days. Most of these newly activated Th cells will then exit the node via the lymph, recirculate through the blood, and re-enter lymph nodes via high endothelial venules. This process of recirculation is fast – it generally takes less than a day – and it is extremely important.

There are four major ingredients that must be "mixed" before the adaptive immune system can produce antibodies: APCs to present antigen to Th cells, Th cells with receptors that recognize the presented antigen, opsonized antigen displayed by follicular dendritic cells, and B cells with receptors that recognize the antigen. Early in an infection, there are not a lot of any of these ingredients around, and naive B and T cells just circulate through the secondary lymphoid organs at random, checking for a match to their receptors. So the probability is pretty small that the rare Th cell that recognizes a particular antigen will arrive at the very same lymph node that is being visited by the rare B cell with specificity for that same antigen. However, if activated Th cells first proliferate to build up their numbers, and then recirculate to lots of lymph nodes and other secondary lymphoid organs, the Th cells with the right stuff get "spread around," so they have a much better chance of encountering those rare B cells that require their help.

When recirculating Th cells enter a node where their cognate antigen is being presented, they will be re-stimulated. Some of the re-stimulated Th cells will proliferate more and recirculate again to spread the help even further. Other re-stimulated Th cells will move to the lymphoid follicles of the lymph node to provide help to needy B cells, and still others will exit the blood to provide cytokine help to warriors doing battle in the tissues.

Killer T cells are also activated in the paracortex of the lymph node if they find their cognate antigen presented by dendritic cells that have been "licensed" by helper T cells. Once activated, CTLs proliferate and recirculate. Some of these CTLs re-enter secondary lymphoid organs and begin this cycle again, whereas others exit the blood at sites of infection to kill virus-infected cells.

B cells also engage in cycles of activation, proliferation, circulation, and re-stimulation, but there are still some mysteries surrounding just where and how virgin B cells are first activated. The most recent evidence indicates that B cells, which have encountered their cognate antigen displayed on follicular dendritic cells, migrate to the border of the lymphoid follicle where they meet activated T cells that have migrated there from the paracortex. It is during this "meeting" that B cells first receive the co-stimulation they require for activation. Both B and T cells then enter the lymphoid follicles, and the B cells proliferate. Many of the newly made B cells exit the lymphoid follicle via the lymph. Some become plasma cells that take up residence in the spleen or bone marrow, where they pump out tons of antibodies. Others recirculate through the lymph and blood and re-enter secondary lymphoid organs. As a result, activated B cells are spread around to many secondary lymphoid organs where, if they are re-stimulated in lymphoid follicles, they can proliferate more and can undergo somatic hypermutation and class switching.

The frantic activity in germinal centers is usually over in about three weeks. By this time, the invader has been repulsed, and most of the opsonized antigen has been "picked" from the dendritic cells by B cells. At this point, most B cells will have left the follicles or will have died there, and the areas that once were germinal centers will look much more like primary lymphoid follicles.

From this discussion, it should be clear that a lymph node is a highly organized place with specific areas for antigen presenting cells, T lymphocytes, and B lymphocytes. But how do APCs and lymphocytes know where to go within a lymph node? In the last few years, immunologists have been busy trying to answer this question, and their experiments have led to the discovery of a special type of cytokine called a "chemokine" (short for chemoattractive cytokine). Although the details are still being worked out, it is known that APCs and lymphocytes, at various stages in their development, express different combinations of receptors for the various members of the chemokine family of proteins. For example, when dendritic cells are activated out in the tissues, they begin to express the chemokine receptor CCR7. This receptor detects a chemokine that is produced by cells in the region of the lymph node where dendritic cells meet T cells. Consequently, once dendritic cells reach a lymph node, they are attracted by the "smell" of this chemokine and go to the correct location. Likewise, follicular dendritic cells in a lymph node produce a chemokine called BLC. B cells express receptors for this chemokine and are attracted to the area of the node where the FDCs are displaying opsonized antigen. Th cells that have been activated by dendritic cells in the T cell areas of the node also express receptors for BLC. When these receptors detect the BLC produced by follicular dendritic cells, the activated (but not the naive) Th cells venture into the B cell areas of the node to aid in the activation of B cells.

Now, of course, human cells don't come equipped with little propellers like some bacteria do, so they can't "swim" in the direction of the source of a chemokine. What human cells do is "crawl." In general terms, the end of the cell that senses the greatest concentration of the cytokine "reaches out" toward the cytokine source, and the other end of the cell is retracted – the rough cellular equivalent of a man crawling toward the scent of a beautiful woman.

In summary, lymph nodes act as "lymph filters" which intercept antigen that arrives from infected tissues either alone or as cargo within a dendritic cell. These nodes provide a concentrated and organized environment of antigen, APCs, T cells, and B cells in which naive B and T cells can be activated, and experienced B and T cells can be re-stimulated. In a lymph node, naive B and T cells can mature into effector cells that produce antibodies (B cells), provide cytokine help (Th cells), and kill infected cells (CTLs). In short, a lymph node can do it all.

As everyone knows, lymph nodes that drain sites of infection tend to swell. For example, if you have a viral infection of your upper respiratory tract (e.g., influenza), the cervical nodes in your neck may become swollen. This swelling is due in part to the proliferation of lymphocytes within the node. In addition, cytokines produced by helper T cells in an active lymph node recruit additional macrophages, which tend to plug up the medullary sinus. As a result, fluid is retained in the node, causing further swelling. When the invader has been defeated, there is no longer sufficient antigen to maintain B and T cells in an activated state. At this point, most B and T cells die from exhaustion or from lack of stimulation, and the swelling in your lymph nodes goes away.

PEYER'S PATCHES

Back in the late seventeenth century, a Swiss anatomist, Johann Peyer, noticed patches of smooth cells embedded in the villi-covered cells that line the small intestine. We now know that these "Peyer's patches" are examples of mucosal associated lymphoid tissues

(MALTs), which function as secondary lymphoid organs. Here is a diagram that shows the basic features of a Peyer's patch:

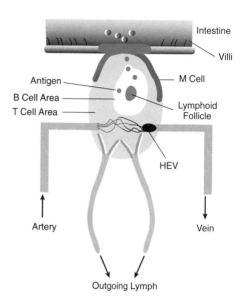

Peyer's patches have high endothelial venules through which lymphocytes can enter from the blood, and, of course, there are outgoing lymphatics that drain lymph away from these tissues. However, unlike lymph nodes, there are no incoming lymphatics that bring lymph into Peyer's patches. So if there are no incoming lymphatics, how does antigen enter this secondary lymphoid organ?

Do you see that smooth cell that crowns the Peyer's patch – the one that doesn't have "hairs" (villi) on it? That cell is called an "M" cell, and it specializes in transporting antigen from the interior (lumen) of the small intestine into the tissues beneath the M cell. To accomplish this, M cells enclose intestinal antigens in vesicles called endosomes that are roughly similar to the phagosomes of macrophages. These endosomes are transported through the M cell, and their contents are then spit out the other side. So, whereas lymph nodes sample antigens from the lymph, Peyer's patches sample antigens from the intestine – and they do it by transporting these antigens through M cells!

Antigen that has been collected by M cells can be carried by the lymph to the lymph nodes that drain the Peyer's patches. Also, if the collected antigen is opsonized by complement or antibodies, it can be captured by follicular dendritic cells in lymphoid follicles that are below the M cells. In fact, except for its unusual method of acquiring antigen, a Peyer's patch is quite similar to a lymph node, with high endothelial venules to bring in T and B cells and special areas where these cells congregate.

Recently it was discovered that M cells are quite selective about the antigens they transport, so M cells don't just take "sips" of whatever is currently in the intestine (how disgusting!). These cells only transport antigens that can bind to molecules on the surface of the M cell. This selectivity makes perfect sense. The whole idea of the M cell and the Peyer's patch is to help initiate an immune response to pathogens that invade via the intestinal tract. But for a pathogen to be troublesome, it has to be able to bind to cells that line the intestines and gain entry into the tissues below. So the minimum requirement for a microbe to be dangerous is that it be able to bind to the surface of an intestinal cell. In contrast, most of the stuff we eat will just pass through the intestine in various stages of digestion without binding to anything. Consequently, by ignoring all the "non-binders," M cells avoid activating the immune system to innocuous food antigens, and concentrate the efforts of the Peyer's patch on potential pathogens.

THE SPLEEN

The final secondary lymphoid organ on our tour is the spleen. This organ is located between an artery and a vein, and it functions as a blood filter. As with Peyer's patches, there are no lymphatics that bring lymph into the spleen. However, in contrast to lymph nodes and Peyer's patches, where entry of B and T cells from the blood occurs only via high endothelial venules, the spleen is like an "open-house party" in which everything in the blood is invited to enter. Here is a schematic diagram of one of the filter units that make up the spleen:

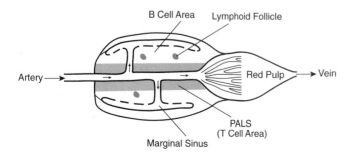

When blood enters from the splenic artery, it is diverted out to the marginal sinuses from which it percolates through the body of the spleen before it is collected into the splenic vein. The marginal sinuses are lined with macrophages that clean up the blood by phagocytosing cell debris and foreign invaders. As they ride along with the blood, naive B cells and T cells are temporarily retained in different areas – T cells in a region called the periarteriolar lymphocyte sheath (PALS) that surrounds the central arteriole, and B cells in the region between the PALS and the marginal sinuses. Once activated by APCs in the PALS, helper T cells move into the lymphoid follicles to give help to B cells that have recognized their cognate antigens – you know the drill.

THE LOGIC OF SECONDARY LYMPHOID ORGANS

By now, I'm sure you have caught on to what Mother Nature is doing here. Each secondary lymphoid organ is strategically positioned to intercept invaders that enter the body by different routes. If the skin is punctured and the tissues becomes infected, an immune response is generated in the lymph nodes that drain those tissues. If you eat contaminated food, an immune response is generated in the Peyer's patches that line your small intestine. If you are invaded by bloodborne pathogens, your spleen is there to filter them out and to initiate an immune response. And if an invader enters via your respiratory tract, another set of secondary lymphoid organs that includes your tonsils is there to defend you.

Not only are the secondary lymphoid organs strategically positioned, they provide a setting that is conducive to the mobilization of weapons that are appropriate to the kinds of invaders they are most likely to encounter. How this works isn't clear yet, but it is believed that the cytokine environments found in different secondary lymphoid organs are different, and that the "resident" cytokines work together with the co-stimulatory molecules provided by APCs to determine the character of the immune response. For example, Peyer's patches specialize in turning out Th cells that secrete a Th2 profile of cytokines as well as B cells that secrete IgA antibodies – weapons that are perfect to defend against intestinal invaders. In contrast, if you are invaded by bacteria from a splinter in your toe, the lymph node behind your knee will produce Th1 cells and B cells that secrete IgG antibodies – weapons ideal for defending against bacteria.

Earlier, I characterized secondary lymphoid organs as "dating bars" where T cells, B cells, and APCs "mingle." Actually, it's even better than that, because secondary lymphoid organs really are more like "dating services." When men and women use a dating service to find a mate, they begin by filling out a questionnaire that gives information on their backgrounds and their goals. Then, a computer goes through all these questionnaires and tries to match up men and women who might be compatible. In this way, the odds of a man finding a woman who is "right" for him is greatly increased, because they have been preselected. This type of preselection also takes place in the secondary lymphoid organs. Here's how it works.

During our tour, we noted that the secondary lymphoid organs are "segregated," with separate areas for naive T cells and B cells. As the billions of Th cells pass through the T cell areas of secondary lymphoid organs, only a tiny fraction of these cells will be activated – those whose cognate antigens are displayed by the antigen presenting cells that also populate the T cell areas. The Th cells that do not find their antigens leave the secondary lymphoid organs and continue to circulate. Only those "lucky" Th cells that are activated in the T cell area will proliferate and then travel to a developing germinal center to provide help to B cells. This makes perfect sense: Allowing useless, non-activated Th cells to enter B cell areas would just clutter things up and would decrease the chances that Th and B cells which are "right" for each other might get together.

Likewise, many B cells enter the B cell areas of secondary lymphoid organs, looking for their cognate antigens displayed by follicular dendritic cells. Most just pass on through, because only a tiny fraction find the antigen that their receptors recognize. These rare B cells are retained in the secondary lymphoid organs and are allowed to interact with activated Th cells. So by preselecting lymphocytes in their respective areas of secondary lymphoid organs, Mother Nature ensures that when Th cells and B cells eventually do meet, they will have the maximum chance of finding their "mates" – just like a dating service!

Although preselecting Th and B cells before they get together is a good idea, the compartmentalization of lymphocytes in the secondary lymphoid organs does raise one problem. Activation of a naive B cell by an activated Th cell involves cell-cell contact during which the CD40L protein on the Th cell binds to the CD40 protein on the B cell. However, while this interaction between CD40L and CD40 is taking place, the engaged CD40L protein is rapidly taken into the interior of the Th cell. Pretty soon, the Th cell doesn't have enough CD40L left on its surface to provide help to B cells. In effect, the Th cell "runs out of gas." To "refill its tank" a Th cell must be re-stimulated. If this occurs, more CD40L proteins will be produced and transported to the surface of the Th cell, and the cell will be back in business. The problem, however, is that when the Th cell runs out of gas, it is no longer in the T cell zone where the APCs that originally provided stimulation reside. So how does the Th cell get re-stimulated?

When B cells bind their cognate antigen displayed on follicular dendritic cells, the antigen is taken into the B cell, cut into fragments, and presented by class II MHC molecules on the B cell surface. And once a B cell has been activated, it will also express B7 proteins on its surface. Consequently, an activated B cell has all the goodies required to function as an APC and to re-stimulate helper T cells that have run out of gas. So, in a lymphoid follicle, Th cells and B cells do a "dance" in which the Th cell provides the co-stimulation (CD40L) required to activate the B cell, and the B cell provides the presented antigen and co-stimulation (B7) required to "re-charge" the T cell.

LYMPHOCYTE TRAFFICKING

So far, we've talked about the secondary lymphoid organs in which B and T cells meet to do their activation thing, but we haven't said much about how these cells know to go there. Immunologists call this process "lymphocyte trafficking." In a human, about 500 billion lymphocytes circulate each day from the blood through the various secondary lymphoid organs and back again to the blood. However, these cells don't just wander around. They follow a carefully orchestrated traffic pattern that maximizes their chances of encountering an invader. Importantly, the traffic patterns of virgin and experienced lymphocytes are different. Let's look first at the travels of a virgin T cell.

T cells begin life in the bone marrow and are educated in the thymus (lots more on this part in the next lecture). When they emerge from the thymus, virgin T cells express on their surfaces a mixture of cellular adhesion molecules that function as "world-wide passports" for travel to any of the secondary lymphoid organs. For example, virgin T cells have a molecule called L-selectin on their surfaces that can bind to its adhesion partner, GlyCAM-1, which is found on the high endothelial venules of lymph nodes. This is their "lymph node passport." Virgin T cells also express the integrin $\alpha4\beta7$, whose adhesion partner, MadCAM-1, is found on the high endothelial venules of Peyer's patches and the lymph nodes that drain the tissues around the intestines (the mesenteric lymph nodes). So this integrin is their passport to the gut region. Equipped with this array of adhesion molecules, inexperienced T cells circulate through all of the secondary lymphoid organs. This makes sense: The genes for a T cell's receptors are assembled by a process of random selection of gene segments – so there is no telling where in the body a given naive T cell will encounter its cognate antigen.

In the secondary lymphoid organs, virgin T cells pass through fields of antigen presenting cells in the T cell areas. If they do not see their cognate antigens advertised there, they re-enter the blood either via the lymph or directly (in the case of the spleen), and continue to recirculate, making a complete circuit every twelve to twenty-four hours. A naive T cell can continue doing this circulation thing for quite some time, but after about six weeks, if the T cell has not encountered its cognate antigen presented by an MHC molecule, it will die by apoptosis, lonely and unsatisfied. In contrast, those lucky naive T cells that do find their antigens are activated in the secondary lymphoid organs. These are now "experienced" T cells.

Experienced T cells also carry passports, but they are "restricted passports," because, during activation, expression of certain adhesion molecules on the T cell surface is increased, while expression of others is decreased. This modulation of cellular adhesion molecule expression is not random – there's a plan here. In fact, the cellular adhesion molecules that activated T cells express depend on where these T cells were activated. For example, T cells activated in a Peyer's patch will express high levels of $\alpha4\beta7$ (the gut-specific integrin), and low levels of L-selectin (the more general, high endothelial venule adhesion molecule). As a result, T cells activated in Peyer's patches tend to return to Peyer's patches. Thus, when activated T cells recirculate, they usually exit the blood and re-enter the same type of secondary lymphoid organ in which they originally encountered antigen. This restricted traffic pattern is quite logical. After all, there is no use having experienced helper T cells recirculate to the lymph node behind your knee if your intestine has been invaded. Certainly not. You want those experienced helper T cells

to get right back to the gut to be re-stimulated and to provide help. So by equipping activated T cells with restricted passports, Mother Nature ensures that these cells will go back to where they are most likely to re-encounter their cognate antigens – be it in a Peyer's patch, a lymph node, or a tonsil.

Now, of course, you don't want T cells to just go round and round. You also want them to exit the blood at sites of infection so they can kill virus-infected cells or provide cytokines that amplify the immune response and recruit even more warriors from the blood. To make this happen, experienced T cells carry additional passports (adhesion molecules) that direct them to exit the blood at places where invaders have started an infection. These T cells employ the same "roll, sniff, stop, exit" technique that neutrophils use to exit the blood into inflamed tissues. For example, T cells that gained their experience in the mucosa express the integrin molecule $\alpha E\beta7$, which just happens to have as its adhesion partner an "addressin" molecule that is expressed on inflamed mucosal blood vessels. As a result, these T cells, which have the right "training" to deal with mucosal invaders, seek out mucosal tissues that have been infected. In these tissues, chemokines given off by the "soldiers" at the front help direct T cells to the battle by binding to chemokine receptors that appeared on the surfaces of the T cells during activation.

In summary, naive T cells have passports that allow them to visit all the secondary lymphoid organs but not sites of inflammation. This traffic pattern brings the entire collection of virgin T cells into contact (in the secondary lymphoid organs) with invaders that may have entered the body at any point, and greatly increases the probability that virgin T cells will be activated. The reason that virgin T cells don't carry passports to battle sites is that they couldn't do anything there anyway – they must be activated first.

In contrast to virgin T cells, experienced T cells have restricted passports that encourage them to return to the same type of secondary lymphoid organ as the one in which they gained their experience. By recirculating preferentially to the kind of organ in which they first encountered antigen, T cells are more likely to be re-stimulated or to find CTLs and B cells that have encountered the same invader and need their help.

Activated T cells also have passports that allow them to exit the blood at sites of infection, enabling CTLs to kill infected cells and Th cells to provide appropriate cytokines to direct the battle. This marvelous "postal system," made up of cellular adhesion molecules and chemokines, insures delivery of the right weapons to the sites where they are needed.

B cell trafficking is roughly similar to T cell trafficking. Like virgin T cells, virgin B cells also have passports that admit them to the complete range of secondary lymphoid organs. However, experienced B cells don't tend to be as migratory as experienced T cells. Most just settle down in secondary lymphoid organs and in the bone marrow, produce antibodies, and let these antibodies do the traveling.

WHY MOTHERS KISS THEIR BABIES

Have you ever wondered why mothers kiss their babies? It's something they all do, you know. Most of the barnyard animals kiss their babies too, although in that case we call it licking. I'm going to tell you why they do it.

The immune system of the newborn human is not very well-developed. In fact, production of IgG antibodies doesn't begin until a few months after birth. Fortunately, IgG antibodies from the mother's blood can cross the placenta into the fetus's blood, so the newborn has this "passive immunity" from the mother to help tide it over. The newborn can also receive another type of passive immunity: IgA antibodies from mother's

milk. During lactation, plasma B cells migrate to the mother's breasts and produce IgA antibodies that are secreted into the milk. This works great, because most pathogens that the baby encounters enter through the mouth and nose, travel to the baby's intestines, and cause diarrhea. By drinking mother's milk that is rich in IgA antibodies, the baby's digestive tract is coated with antibodies that can intercept these pathogens.

When you think about it, however, a mother has been exposed to many different pathogens during her life, and the antibodies she makes to most of them will not be of any use to the infant. For example, it is likely that the mother has antibodies which recognize the Epstein-Barr virus that causes mononucleosis, but babies probably won't be exposed to this virus until they start kissing. So wouldn't it be great if the mother could somehow provide antibodies that recognize those pathogens that the baby is encountering – and not provide antibodies that the baby has no use for? Well, that's exactly what happens.

When a mother kisses her baby, she "samples" those pathogens that are on the baby's face – the ones the baby is about to ingest. These samples are taken up by the mother's secondary lymphoid organs (e.g., her tonsils), and memory B cells specific for those pathogens are re-stimulated. These activated B cells then traffic to the mother's breasts where they produce a ton of antibodies – the very antibodies that the baby needs!

THOUGHT QUESTIONS

1. What are the functions of the secondary lymphoid organs?

2. Make a table for each of the secondary lymphoid organs we discussed (lymph node, Peyer's patch, spleen) that lists how antigen, T cells, and B cells enter and leave these organs.

3. In the T cell areas of secondary lymphoid organs, activated dendritic cells and Th cells interact. What goes on during this "dance"?

4. In the lymphoid follicles of secondary lymphoid organs, B cells and Th cells interact. What goes on during this "dance"?

5. What is the advantage of having <u>virgin</u> T cells circulate through all the secondary lymphoid organs?

6. What is the advantage of having <u>activated</u> T cells circulate through selected secondary lymphoid organs?

7. Why are virgin T cells not allowed out into the tissues, and what keeps them from going there?

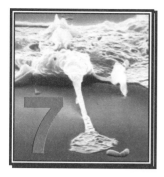

TOLERANCE INDUCTION AND MHC RESTRICTION

REVIEW

In the last lecture, we talked in some detail about three representative secondary lymphoid organs: a lymph node, a Peyer's patch, and the spleen. B and T cells enter lymph nodes from the blood (by passing between specialized high endothelial cells) or via the lymph. Antigen and APCs bearing antigen enter lymph nodes via lymph that drains from tissues, so this organ functions as a lymph filter that intercepts invaders. In contrast, antigen is transported into the Peyer's patches through specialized M cells that sample antigen from the intestine. This antigen can either interact with B and T cells that have entered the Peyer's patches via high endothelial venules or it can travel with the lymph to lymph nodes that drain the Peyer's patch. Thus, the Peyer's patch is a secondary lymphoid organ that is designed to deal with pathogens attempting to breach the intestinal mucosal barrier. Finally, we talked about the spleen, a secondary lymphoid organ that is quite different from either a lymph node or a Peyer's patch in that it has no incoming lymphatics and no high endothelial venules. As a result of this "plumbing," antigen and lymphocytes must enter the spleen via the blood. This construction makes the spleen an ideal blood filter that intercepts bloodborne pathogens.

So secondary lymphoid organs are strategically situated to intercept invaders that breach the physical barriers and enter the tissues and the blood. Because of their location, they play a critical role in immunity by creating an environment in which antigen, antigen presenting cells, and lymphocytes can gather to initiate an immune response. Virgin helper T cells travel though the blood, and under the influence of adhesion molecules and chemokines, enter the secondary lymphoid organs. If a Th cell does not encounter its cognate antigen displayed by an APC in the T cell

zone, it exits the organ via lymph or blood, and visits other secondary lymphoid organs in search of its antigen. On the other hand, if during its visit to a secondary lymphoid organ, a Th cell does find its cognate antigen displayed by class II MHC molecules on a dendritic cell, it becomes activated and proliferates. Most of the progeny exit the secondary lymphoid organ and travel through the lymph and the blood. These "experienced" Th cells have adhesion molecules on their surfaces that encourage them to re-enter the same type of secondary lymphoid organ in which they were activated (e.g., a Peyer's patch or a peripheral lymph node). This recirculation following initial activation and proliferation spreads the activated Th cells around to the more than a thousand secondary lymphoid organs where B cells or CTLs may be waiting for their help. Recirculating Th cells also can exit the blood vessels that run through sites of inflammation. There the Th cells amplify the immune response by providing cytokines that strengthen the reaction of the innate and adaptive systems to the invader, and which recruit even more immune system cells from the blood.

Virgin CTLs also circulate through the blood, lymph, and secondary lymphoid organs. They can be activated if they encounter their cognate antigen displayed by class I MHC molecules on the surfaces of antigen presenting cells in the T cell zones of secondary lymphoid organs. Like Th cells, they can proliferate and recirculate to secondary lymphoid organs to be re-stimulated, or they can leave the circulation and enter inflamed tissues to kill cells infected with viruses or other parasites.

Virgin B cells also travel to secondary lymphoid organs like lymph nodes and Peyer's patches looking for their cognate antigens. If they are unsuccessful, they continue circulating through the blood, lymph, and secondary lymphoid organs until they either find their cognate antigens or die of neglect. In the lymphoid follicles of the secondary lymphoid organs, the lucky B cell that finds the antigen to which its receptors can bind will migrate to the border of the lymphoid follicle. There, if it receives the required co-stimulation from an activated helper T cell, the B cell will be activated, and will proliferate to produce many more B cells with the same antigen specificity.

All this activity converts a primary lymphoid follicle, which is just a loose collection of follicular dendritic cells and B cells, into a "germinal center" in which B cells proliferate and mature. In a germinal center, B cells may "class switch" to produce IgA, IgG, or IgE antibodies, and they may undergo somatic hypermutation to increase the average affinity of their receptors for antigen. Most of these B cells become plasma cells and travel to the spleen, bone marrow, or secondary lymphoid organs, where they produce antibodies. Others recirculate to secondary lymphoid organs that are similar to the one in which they were activated. There they amplify the response by being re-stimulated to proliferate some more. Still other B cells go back to the resting state in the spleen or bone marrow to function as memory cells.

In summary, virgin B and T cells are equipped with adhesion molecules and chemokine receptors that promote travel to all secondary lymphoid organs, but which do not allow travel to inflamed tissues. As a result, the entire repertoire of TCRs and BCRs is brought together in secondary lymphoid organs – where the probability is highest that they will encounter their cognate antigens in an environment appropriate for activation. Once activated, B and T cells receive restricted passports to travel back to the same type of secondary lymphoid organ in which they were originally activated, and to exit the blood at sites of infection so that they can participate in the struggle against invaders.

SELF TOLERANCE AND MHC RESTRICTION

The subject of this lecture is one of the most exciting in all of immunology. Part of that excitement arises because, although a huge amount of research has been done on tolerance and MHC restriction, there are still many unanswered questions. What really makes this topic so exciting, however, is that it is so important. B cells and T cells must "learn" not to recognize our own "self" antigens as dangerous, for otherwise we would all die of autoimmune disease. In addition, T cells must be "restricted" to recognize self MHC, so that the attention of T cells will be focused on MHC-peptide complexes and not on unpresented antigen. Indeed, Nobel Prizes await the immunologists who finally discover how T cells are taught these two important lessons.

Perhaps the major problem in understanding tolerance and MHC restriction is that it is technically very difficult to follow T cells around as they are educated. What you'd like to do is to introduce a model "self" antigen into an animal (mice are quite popular), and observe how T cells that have receptors for this antigen are tolerized or restricted. However, because T cell receptors are so diverse, only a tiny fraction of the T cells in a mouse will have receptors that recognize a given antigen. So following those rare T cells around in the crowd of T cells that don't recognize your favorite antigen is really tough.

To increase the number of T cells that respond to a given antigen, two methods have been devised, neither of which is without flaws. The first method involves the use of "superantigens." These are proteins that cause the activation of a relatively large fraction (usually 5% to 25%) of the helper T cells in a mouse. There are two sources of superantigens: toxins produced by bacteria and proteins encoded by viruses. In both cases, superantigens work by binding to the variable region of the TCR and to the class II MHC molecule, "clamping" them together.

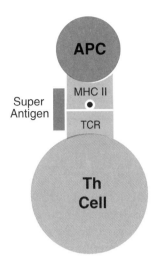

This superantigen "clamp" makes the binding between the MHC molecule and the TCR so strong that essentially every T cell that happens to have this particular variable region will be activated. As you can imagine, having 25% of your Th cells activated all at once might be a problem. Indeed, the superantigen encoded by a common bacterium, *Staphylococcus aureus*, can cause toxic shock syndrome and food poisoning by hyperactivating the immune system. Although superantigens were all the rage a few years ago, this tool is less popular now, because immunologists recognize that the way a T cell receptor interacts with a superantigen is quite different from the "normal" interaction between TCR and MHC-peptide that we have discussed in earlier lectures.

The second tool immunologists have used to follow T cells around is a mouse that makes TCRs with only one specificity. Transgenic mouse technology has progressed to the point where you can now wipe out just about any gene you wish and replace it with another one. All you need are lots of mice and lots of money. Anyway, what immunologists have done is to insert into the chromosomes of a mouse a pre-assembled TCR gene that recognizes some particular protein (e.g., a protein from a chicken) presented by either the mouse's class I or class II MHC molecules. This transgenic mouse is then mated with a mutant mouse that cannot assemble its own TCR genes. The result is a mouse that only makes T cells with TCRs that recognize the chicken protein. This isn't all that great for the mouse, but it certainly makes it much easier to follow these T cells through their education process. However, as you will see during this lecture, the number of TCRs that a T cell expresses on its surface changes with time as the cell matures and is educated. So far, the TCRs in these transgenic mice don't behave that way. They are

expressed at a particular stage of development and at a certain level and that's it. So when interpreting an experiment that uses these mice, you have to ask whether the results that are obtained might be influenced by the timing and the level of TCR expression.

THE THYMUS

T cells first learn tolerance of self in the thymus, a small organ located just below the neck. This process is usually called "central tolerance induction." Here's how immunologists view the thymus:

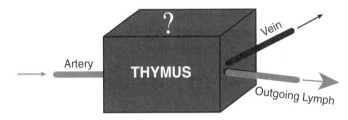

As you can see, the thymus is a very mysterious organ. Like the spleen, the thymus has no incoming lymphatics, so cells enter the thymus from the blood. However, in contrast to the spleen, which welcomes anything that is in the blood, entry of cells into the thymus is quite restricted, although immunologists don't know yet what "password" is needed for entry. Immature T cells from the bone marrow are presumed to enter the thymus from the blood, somewhere in the middle of the thymus. However, exactly how this happens is not understood, because the high endothelial cells that allow lymphocytes to exit the blood into secondary lymphoid organs are missing from the thymus. Antigens are also thought to enter from the blood, but again, the rules that govern their entry are unclear.

What is known is that the T cells which enter the thymus from the bone marrow are "nude": They don't express CD4, CD8, or a TCR. These cells first make their way to the outer region of the thymus (the cortex) and begin to proliferate.

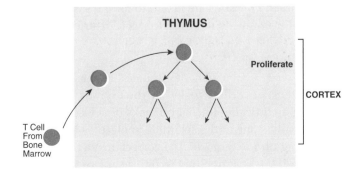

About this time, some of the cells start to rearrange the gene segments that encode the β and α chains of the TCR. If these rearrangements are successful, the T cell begins to express low levels of the TCR and its associated, accessory proteins (the CD3 protein complex). As a result, these formerly nude cells are soon "dressed" with CD4, CD8, and TCR molecules on their surfaces. Because all of these T cells express both CD4 and CD8 co-receptor molecules, they are called "double positive" (DP) cells.

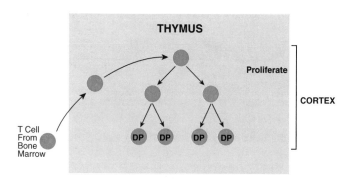

During this "reverse striptease," another important change takes place. When the T cell was nude, it was resistant to death by apoptosis, because it expressed no Fas antigen (which can trigger death when ligated) and it expressed high levels of Bcl-2 (a cellular protein that protects against apoptosis). In contrast, in the double-positive state, the T cell expresses high levels of Fas on its surface and it produces very little Bcl-2. Consequently, it is exquisitely sensitive to signals that can trigger death by apoptosis. It is in this highly vulnerable condition that the T cell will be tested for tolerance of self and MHC restriction. If it fails either test, it will be killed.

MHC RESTRICTION

Immunologists still are not sure of the order in which these two exams are taken, so for the sake of discussion, I'll assume that the test for MHC restriction precedes the exam for tolerance of self. The process of testing T cells for MHC restriction is usually referred to as "positive selection." The "examiners" here are epithelial cells in the cortical region of the thymus, and the question a cortical epithelial cell asks of a T cell is: Do you recognize one of the self MHC molecules that I am expressing on my surface? The correct answer is, "Yes, I do!" for if the TCR does not recognize any of these self MHC molecules, the T cell dies.

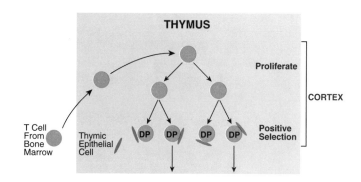

When I say "self" MHC, I simply mean those MHC molecules that are expressed by the person (or mouse) who "owns" this thymus. Yes, this does seem like a no brainer – that my T cells would be tested in my thymus on my MHC molecules – but immunologists like to emphasize this point by saying "self MHC."

The MHC molecules on the surface of the cortical epithelial cells are actually loaded with peptides, so what a TCR really recognizes is the combination of a self MHC molecule and its associated peptide. These peptides represent a "sampling" of the proteins that are being made by the thymic cells (displayed by class I MHC molecules) plus a "sampling" of all the proteins that the thymic cells have picked up from the tissues of the thymus (displayed by class II MHC molecules).

THE LOGIC OF MHC RESTRICTION

Let's pause here for a moment between exams to ask an important question: Why do T cells need to be tested to be sure that they can recognize peptides presented by self MHC molecules? After all, most humans complete their lifetimes without ever seeing "foreign" MHC molecules (e.g., on a transplanted organ), so MHC restriction can't involve discriminating between your MHC molecules and mine. No, MHC restriction has nothing to do with foreign vs. self – it's all about "focus." As we discussed in Lecture 4, we want the system to be set up so that T cells focus on antigens that are presented by MHC molecules. However, T cell receptors are made by mixing and matching gene segments, so they are incredibly diverse. As a result, it is certain that in the collection of TCRs expressed on T cells, there will be many which recognize unpresented antigens, just as a B cell's receptors do. These T cells must be eliminated. Otherwise the wonderful system of antigen presentation by MHC molecules won't work. So the reason positive selection (MHC restriction) is so important is that it sets up a system in which all mature

T cells will have TCRs that recognize antigens presented by MHC molecules.

CENTRAL TOLERANCE INDUCTION

Those lucky T cells which have TCRs that can recognize self MHC plus peptide proceed to the second test in the thymus: tolerance of self. This exam is frequently referred to as "negative selection." The cells that administer this test are different from those that test for positive selection. Whereas the positively selecting cells are "real" thymus cells that have been present in the thymus since embryonic development, the negatively selecting cells are dendritic cells that have migrated to the thymus from the bone marrow. Although thymic DCs have the starfish-like shape that is characteristic of dendritic cells in general, they are different from either the antigen presenting dendritic cells or the follicular dendritic cells we discussed previously. Thymic dendritic cells congregate mainly in the central region of the thymus called the "medulla."

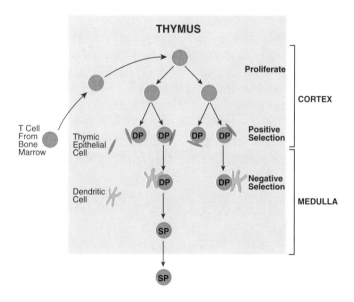

The exam question posed by a thymic dendritic cell is, "Do you recognize any of the self peptides displayed by the MHC molecules on my surface?" The correct answer is, "No," for T cells with receptors that do recognize the combination of MHC molecules and self peptides are killed. The reason this second test, which eliminates T cells that could react against our own "self" antigens, is so important is that if such self-reactive T cells were not eliminated, autoimmune disease could result. For example, Th cells that recognized self antigens could help B cells make antibodies

that would tag our own molecules (e.g., the insulin proteins in our blood) for destruction. In addition, CTLs could be produced that would attack our own cells.

One important feature of negative selection is that the cells which administer the exam, the thymic dendritic cells, survive for only a few days in the thymus. Consequently, they only present what you might call "current" self antigen. This is really smart, because if foreign antigens were to reach the thymus (as they certainly can during an infection), dendritic cells could take up these antigens and use them for testing, just as if they were authentic "self" antigens. As a result, any maturing T cells that recognized the invader would be "deleted" for as long as thymic dendritic cells continued to present the foreign antigens. The short lifetime of thymic dendritic cells protects against this possibility and allows T cells to be examined only on "new material." Once foreign antigens associated with an infection have been eliminated from the body, freshly made dendritic cells will no longer present foreign antigen as self – and T cells that can recognize the invader will again survive negative selection.

The final result of all this testing is a T cell with receptors that <u>do</u> recognize self MHC-peptide complexes presented by thymic epithelial cells, but which do <u>not</u> recognize self antigens presented by MHC molecules on thymic dendritic cells. Most students are not too thrilled about exams that last more than an hour, so I thought you might be interested to know that together these two tests take about two weeks! We're talking major exams here, where the life of each T cell hangs in the balance.

The "thymic graduates" that pass these tests express high levels (i.e., many molecules) of the T cell receptor on their surfaces, and either the CD4 or CD8 co-receptor, but not both. Consequently, they are called "single positive" (SP) cells. Each day in the thymus of a young person, about 60 million double positive cells are tested, but only about 2 million single positive cells exit the thymus – so roughly 3% of the "candidates" pass these exams. The rest die a horrible death by apoptosis, and are quickly eaten by macrophages in the thymus.

THE RIDDLE OF MHC RESTRICTION AND TOLERANCE INDUCTION

Now, if you've been paying close attention, you may be wondering how <u>any</u> T cells could possibly pass both exams. After all, to pass the test for MHC restriction, their TCRs must be able to recognize MHC plus self peptide. Yet, to pass the tolerance exam, their TCRs must not be able to recognize MHC plus self peptide. Doesn't it seem that the two exams should cancel each other out, allowing no T cells to pass? It certainly does, and this is the essence of the riddle of self tolerance: How can the same T cell receptor possibly mediate both positive selection (MHC restriction) and negative selection (tolerance induction)? In fact, it is even more complicated than that because once T cells have been educated in the thymus, their TCRs must then be able to signal activation when they encounter invaders presented by MHC molecules. So the question that vexes immunologists is: How does the same TCR, when it engages MHC-peptide complexes, signal three very different outcomes – positive selection, negative selection, or activation?

Unfortunately, I can't answer this riddle (otherwise I'd be on my way to Sweden), but I can tell you the current thinking. Immunologists believe that the events leading to MHC restriction and tolerance induction are similar to those involved in the activation of T cells: cell-cell adhesion, TCR clustering, and co-stimulation. It is hypothesized that in the thymus, positive selection (survival) of T cells with receptors that recognize self MHC results from a relatively weak interaction between TCRs and MHC-self peptide displayed on thymic epithelial cells. Negative selection (death) is induced by a strong interaction between TCRs and MHC-self peptide expressed on bone marrow–derived, thymic dendritic cells. Activation of T cells after they leave the thymus results from a strong interaction between TCRs and MHC-peptide displayed by professional antigen presenting cells.

The question, of course, is what makes the effect of these three interactions of MHC-peptide with a T cell receptor so different – life, death, or activation. One key element appears to be the properties of the cell that "sends" the signal. In the case of MHC restriction, this is a thymic epithelial cell. For tolerance induction, the cell is a bone marrow–derived dendritic cell. For activation, the "sender" is a specialized antigen presenting cell. These cells are very different, and it is likely that they differ in the cellular adhesion molecules they express, and in the number of MHC-peptide complexes they display on their surfaces. These differences could dramatically influence the "strength" of the signal that is sent through the T cell receptor. In addition, these three cell types are likely to express different mixtures of co-stimulatory molecules – and co-stimulatory signals could change the meaning of the signal that results from TCR-MHC-peptide engagements.

Not only are the cells that send the signals different, but the "receiver" (the T cell) also may change between exams. It is known that the number of TCRs on the surface of the T cell increases as the cell is educated, and it is also possible that the "wiring" within the T cell changes as the T cell matures. These differences in TCR density and signal processing could influence the interpretation of the signals sent by the three types of sender cells.

Although many of the pieces of the MHC restriction/tolerance induction puzzle probably have been found, immunologists still have not been able to assemble them into a consistent story. It is very likely, however, that this important riddle will soon be solved.

TOLERANCE BY IGNORANCE

Thankfully, most T cells with receptors that could recognize our own proteins are eliminated in the thymus. However, central tolerance is not foolproof. If it were, every single T cell would have to be tested on every possible self antigen in the thymus – and that's a lot to ask. The probability is great that T cells with receptors which have a high affinity for self antigens that are abundant in the thymus will be deleted there. However, T cells with receptors that have a low affinity for self antigens, or that recognize self antigens rarely found in the thymus are less likely to be negatively selected – they may just slip through the "cracks" of central tolerance induction. Fortunately, the system has been set up to deal with this possibility.

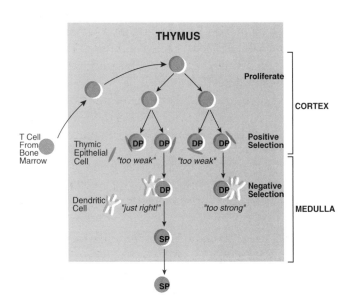

Virgin T cells circulate through the secondary lymphoid organs, but are not allowed out into the tissues. This traffic pattern takes these virgins to the areas of the body where they are most likely to encounter APCs and become activated. However, the travel restriction that keeps virgin T cells out of the tissues also is important in maintaining self tolerance. The reason is that, as a rule, those self antigens that are abundant in the secondary lymphoid organs where virgin lymphocytes are activated are also abundant in the place where T cells are tolerized, the thymus. Therefore, as a result of the traffic pattern followed by virgin T cells, most T cells that could be activated by abundant self antigens found in secondary lymphoid organs will already have been eliminated by seeing that same abundant self antigen in the thymus.

In contrast, T cells whose receptors recognize antigens that are relatively rare in the thymus may escape deletion there. However, these same antigens are usually present at such low concentrations in the secondary lymphoid organs that APCs there will have too few MHC-peptide complexes on their surfaces to activate T cells. Thus, although rare self antigens are present in the secondary lymphoid organs, and although T cells have receptors that can recognize them, these T cells remain functionally "ignorant" of their presence, because the antigens are too rare to trigger activation. So lymphocyte traffic patterns play a key role not only in ensuring the efficient activation of the adaptive immune system, but also in preserving tolerance to self antigens.

PERIPHERAL TOLERANCE

Of course, virgin T cells aren't perfect, and some do stray from the prescribed traffic pattern and venture out into the tissues. There these "lawbreaker" cells may encounter self antigens that were too rare in the thymus to trigger deletion, but which are abundant enough in the tissues to activate these T cells. For example, there are "organ-specific" self antigens that are abundant in the heart or the kidney, but which usually are not present at any appreciable level in the thymus. To deal with this situation, there is a third level of protection against autoimmunity – peripheral tolerance.

Because of the two-key requirement for T cell activation, virgin T cells must not only encounter enough presented antigen to cluster their receptors,

but they must also receive co-stimulatory signals from the cell that is presenting the antigen. That's where antigen presenting cells come in. These special cells have lots of MHC molecules on their surfaces to present antigens, and they also express co-stimulatory molecules like B7. In contrast, "ordinary cells" like heart and kidney cells generally don't express high levels of MHC proteins or don't express co-stimulatory molecules, or both. As a result, a virgin T cell with receptors that recognize a kidney antigen could probably go right up to a kidney cell and not be activated by it. In fact, it's even better than that. When a T cell recognizes its cognate antigen on a cell, but does not receive the appropriate co-stimulatory signals, that T cell is "neutered." It looks like a T cell, but it can no longer perform. Immunologists say the cell is "anergized." In many cases, cells that are anergized eventually die, so peripheral tolerance induction can result in either anergy or death (deletion). Consequently, the requirement for the second, co-stimulatory "key" during T cell activation protects us against virgin T cells that venture outside their normal traffic pattern.

TOLERANCE DUE TO ACTIVATION-INDUCED DEATH

Okay, so what if a T cell escapes deletion in the thymus, breaks the traffic laws, and ventures out into the tissues? And what if this T cell just happens to find its cognate antigen displayed by MHC molecules at a high enough density to crosslink its receptors on a cell that just happens to be able to provide the co-stimulation required to activate the T cell? What then? Well, all is not lost, because there is yet another "layer" of tolerance induction that can protect us in this unlikely situation. It is called activation-induced cell death. Here's how it works.

Once an invader has been vanquished, it is very important that mechanisms exist which will turn the immune response off. For example, once an invader has been vanquished, most T cells die off because no antigens are left in the body to stimulate them. This is one way that "leftover" T cells can be eliminated. But there is another way that T cells can be deleted when they no longer are needed.

CTLs have Fas ligand proteins prominently displayed on their surfaces, and one way they kill is by plugging this protein into its binding partner, Fas, which is present on the surfaces of target cells. When these proteins connect, the target is triggered to commit suicide by apoptosis. Virgin T cells are "wired" so that they are insensitive to ligation of their Fas proteins. However, when these T cells are activated and then reactivated many times during an attack, their internal wiring changes and they become increasingly more sensitive to ligation of their Fas proteins, either by their own Fas ligand proteins or by Fas ligand proteins on other T cells. This makes these "old" T cells targets for Fas-mediated killing – either by suicide or by "homicide." Immunologists call this activation-induced cell death. Getting rid of old T cells by activation-induced cell death makes perfect sense. After all, most invasions by viruses or bacteria result in acute infections that either are quickly dealt with by the immune system (in a matter of days or weeks) or that overwhelm the immune system and kill you. So there really is no reason to have activated T cells survive for a long period to deal with an acute infection.

In addition to providing a mechanism to get rid of worn-out T cells, activation-induced cell death also helps protect against virgin T cells that break the traffic rules and are activated by self antigens out in the tissues. T cells in this situation are stimulated over and over by the ever-present self antigens, and when this happens, the self-reactive T cells usually are eliminated by activation-induced cell death. It is as if the immune system senses that this continuous reactivation "ain't natural," and does away with the offending, self-reactive T cells.

In summary, induction of T cell tolerance is multi-layered. No single mechanism of tolerance induction is 100% efficient, but because there are multiple mechanisms, autoimmune diseases are relatively rare. T cells with receptors which recognize antigens that are abundant in the secondary lymphoid organs usually are efficiently deleted in the thymus. Self antigens that are rare enough in the thymus to allow self-reactive T cells to escape deletion usually are also too rare to activate virgin T cells in the secondary lymphoid organs. Thus, because of their restricted traffic pattern, virgin T cells normally remain functionally ignorant of self antigens that are rare in the thymus. In those cases where virgin T cells do venture outside the blood-lymph-secondary lymphoid organ system, they generally encounter tissue-specific antigens in a context that leads to anergy or death, not activation. Finally, those rare T cells that are activated by recognizing self antigens in the tissues usually die from chronic re-stimulation.

B CELL TOLERANCE

Immunologists once thought that it might not be necessary to delete B cells with receptors that recognize self antigens. The idea was that, because the T cells needed to "help" these potentially self-reactive B cells would already have been killed or anergized, B cell tolerance would be "covered" by T cell tolerance. However, as it became clear that B cells could sometimes be activated without T cell help, it was realized that there must be mechanisms for tolerizing B cells. Although B cell tolerance is not as well studied as T cell tolerance, there do seem to be many similarities between tolerance induction in B and T cells.

It is now believed that B cells can be tolerized where they are born – in the bone marrow. This would be the B cell equivalent of central tolerance induction. After B cells mix and match gene segments to construct the final genes for their receptors, they are "tested" to see if these receptors recognize self antigens that are present in the bone marrow. If its receptors do recognize a self antigen, a B cell is given another chance to rearrange its light chain gene and come up with new receptors that don't recognize self antigens. This process is called "receptor editing." Although the details of how receptor editing works are not yet understood, it appears that at least 25% of all B cells take advantage of this "second chance." Finally, those B cells with receptors that do not bind to self antigens are released from the bone marrow, and the others, whose receptors do recognize self antigens, are killed.

Of course, induction of B cell tolerance in the bone marrow has the same problems as T cell tolerance induction in the thymus: B cells with receptors that recognize self antigens that are rare in the marrow can slip through the cracks. Fortunately, bone marrow mostly contains the same abundant self antigens that are found in the secondary lymphoid organs where virgin B cells will be activated. Consequently, self antigens that are too rare to efficiently delete B cells in the bone marrow usually are too rare to activate these B cells in the secondary lymphoid organs. So the traffic pattern of virgin B cells, which restricts them to circulating through the secondary lymphoid organs, helps "protect" them from encountering abundant self antigens that are not present in the bone marrow.

There are also mechanisms that can tolerize B cells that do break the traffic laws. For example, virgin B cells that venture into the tissues can be anergized or deleted if they recognize their cognate antigen but do not receive T cell help. In addition, B cells that are chronically stimulated by self antigens eventually die by apoptosis. Thus, B cells are subject to mechanisms which enforce self tolerance that are similar, but probably not identical, to those which tolerize T cells outside the thymus.

MAINTENANCE OF B CELL TOLERANCE IN GERMINAL CENTERS

You may be wondering whether B cells undergoing somatic hypermutation might end up with receptors that can recognize self antigens. If they did, these B cells could produce antibodies that would cause autoimmune disease. Fortunately, it turns out that this usually doesn't happen, and the reasons are quite interesting.

B cells in germinal centers are very "fragile." Unless they receive "rescue" signals, they die by apoptosis. In this sense, germinal center B cells resemble the fragile T cells that undergo MHC restriction and tolerance induction in the thymus. The signals required to rescue B cells from death in the germinal center are the same as those required to activate B cells in the first place: recognition of cognate antigen in a form that crosslinks BCRs, and co-stimulatory signals from helper T cells. B cells seem to need these two rescue signals more or less continuously while they are in the germinal center.

If a B cell hypermutates in a germinal center so that its receptors recognize a self antigen, it is very unlikely to find (and be rescued by) that self antigen advertised on follicular dendritic cells. After all, FDCs only display antigens that have been opsonized – and self antigens usually aren't opsonized. What's more, experiments indicate that for a B cell to be rescued from death in a germinal center, not only must its BCRs be crosslinked by antigen, but its complement receptors (which function as co-receptors) must also engage complement fragments that are opsonizing the antigen. This double requirement for BCR <u>and</u> complement receptor crosslinking probably explains why humans who lack a functional complement system do not have germinal centers.

So the first problem that self-reactive B cells face in the germinal center is the lack of complement-opsonized self antigen on follicular dendritic cells. But they have another problem – lack of co-stimulation – and the reason for this is even more interesting. After Th cells have been activated in the T cell zones of secondary lymphoid organs, they move to lymphoid follicles to give help to B cells. This help takes place during a "dance" in which the Th cell and the B cell stimulate each other. While dancing, the Th cell provides the CD40L needed to co-stimulate the B cell. In return, the activated B cell satisfies the helper cell's needs by supplying B7 co-stimulation, and by using its class II MHC molecules to present fragments of its cognate antigen to the Th cell. The subtle but important point here is that for this mutual activation thing between a B cell and a T cell to work, these cells must be looking at parts of the same antigen. So if the B cell hypermutates so that its BCRs bind to and present a different antigen (e.g., a self antigen), that new antigen will not be the Th cell's cognate antigen. As a result, the B and T cells will not be able to cooperate to keep each other stimulated. They will have lost their "common interest," and dancing together will be out of the question.

Because B cells require T cell help to survive in the germinal center, the interdependence of B and T cells keeps B cells "on track" as they undergo somatic hypermutation. Consequently, self tolerance is preserved during B cell hypermutation for two reasons: the lack of complement-opsonized self antigen required for efficient BCR signaling, and the lack of germinal center Th cells, which can provide help for B cells that recognize self antigen.

A SUMMARY FIGURE

T cell tolerance is a multilayered process in which several "levels" of tolerance-inducing mechanisms insure that, for most humans, autoimmunity never happens.

EPILOGUE

At this point you should have a good overall view of how the immune system is designed to work in healthy individuals. In the next two lectures, we will explore the roles that the immune system plays in disease.

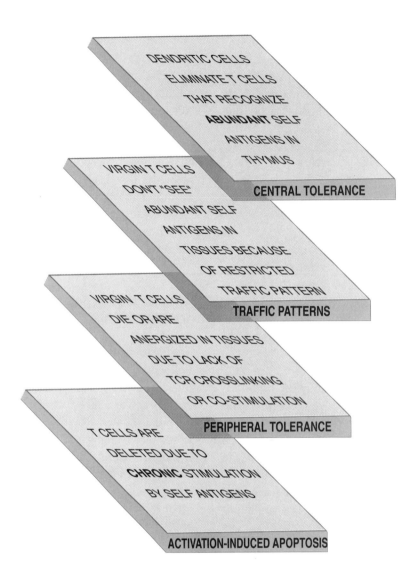

DENDRITIC CELLS ELIMINATE T CELLS THAT RECOGNIZE **ABUNDANT** SELF ANTIGENS IN THYMUS — **CENTRAL TOLERANCE**

VIRGIN T CELLS DON'T "SEE" ABUNDANT SELF ANTIGENS IN TISSUES BECAUSE OF RESTRICTED TRAFFIC PATTERN — **TRAFFIC PATTERNS**

VIRGIN T CELLS DIE OR ARE ANERGIZED IN TISSUES DUE TO LACK OF TCR CROSSLINKING OR CO-STIMULATION — **PERIPHERAL TOLERANCE**

T CELLS ARE DELETED DUE TO **CHRONIC** STIMULATION BY SELF ANTIGENS — **ACTIVATION-INDUCED APOPTOSIS**

THOUGHT QUESTIONS

1. Why is it important that T cells be tested to be sure they can recognize self MHC molecules? Wouldn't it be a lot simpler just to eliminate this exam?

2. For T cells being educated in the thymus, what is the functional definition of self (i.e., what do these T cells consider to be self or non-self peptides)?

3. What is the underlying difficulty in a T cell satisfying both the requirement for MHC restriction (posi-tive selection) and the requirement for tolerance of self (negative selection)?

4. Why are mechanisms needed that can tolerize T cells once they leave the thymus?

5. Explain why the traffic pattern of virgin T cells plays a role in maintaining tolerance of self.

6. Why is it important that B cells also be taught tolerance of self?

Part II

The Immune System in Disease

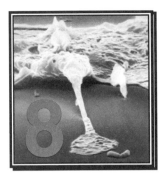

IMMUNOPATHOLOGY: THE IMMUNE SYSTEM GONE WRONG

REVIEW

In the last lecture, we discussed what is probably the most important riddle left to be solved by immunologists: How can the same T cell receptor mediate positive selection (MHC restriction), negative selection (tolerance induction), and activation? This riddle has not been solved, but here's the current thinking.

In the thymus, positive selection (survival) of T cells with receptors that recognize self MHC results from a relatively weak interaction between TCRs and MHC-self peptides displayed on thymic epithelial cells. This weak interaction is enough to focus the attention of T cells on antigens presented by MHC molecules, insuring that recognition is restricted to presented antigens, not "native" antigens. Negative selection (death) of cells with TCRs that recognize self antigens in the thymus is induced by a strong interaction between TCRs and MHC-self peptides expressed on bone marrow–derived, thymic dendritic cells. Finally, activation of T cells after they leave the thymus results from a strong interaction between TCRs and MHC-peptides displayed by professional antigen presenting cells.

The important point here is that the interactions that lead to these three very different outcomes are between the TCR and MHC-peptides displayed by three very different types of cells. These cells can be expected to express different adhesion molecules, different co-stimulatory molecules, and even different cytokines – so the outcome of each of these interactions probably depends, at least in part, on the cell type with which the T cell interacts. In addition, T cells may learn from experience: Their internal "wiring" may change as they are educated and mature. Consequently, as T cells grow up, the same

signals may be processed differently and may produce different outcomes.

Although the mechanisms involved are not completely understood, the end result of the thymic experience is that only about 3% of the T cells that enter selection exit from the thymus. These lucky T cells have receptors which do not recognize peptides derived from self antigens that are relatively abundant in the thymus. Of course, many T cells that exit the thymus have receptors which will recognize foreign peptides presented by MHC – that's the whole idea of this game – but some of them also have receptors which recognize relatively rare self antigens that are not abundant enough in the thymus to efficiently delete T cells. So although thymic (central) tolerance induction is pretty good, it isn't the whole story. To take care of T cells that slip through thymic selection, several forms of "remedial education" exist outside the thymus that back up thymic tolerance induction.

One way of dealing with T cells that escape deletion in the thymus is to restrict the trafficking of virgin T cells to blood, lymph, and secondary lymphoid organs. Most self antigens that are abundant in the secondary lymphoid organs, where T cells are activated, also are abundant in the thymus. Consequently, T cells that could be activated by these self antigens already will have been deleted in the thymus. On the other hand, self antigens that are not abundant enough in the thymus to efficiently delete T cells usually are present in secondary lymphoid organs at concentrations too low to activate potentially self-reactive T cells. Therefore, because of their restricted traffic pattern, most virgin T cells with TCRs that could recognize rare self antigens remain functionally ignorant of their existence, simply because they don't encounter enough of these antigens during their travels.

Of course, not all virgin T cells are law-abiding, and some will leave their normal circulation pattern and wind up in the tissues. To deal with these "law breakers," Mother Nature has a few more tricks up her sleeve. For T cells to be activated, they must recognize their cognate MHC-peptide combination at a high enough concentration to trigger activation. Fortunately, most cells in the tissues don't express high enough levels of MHC-peptide to activate naive T cells. In addition, to be activated, virgin T cells must receive co-stimulatory signals from the cell that presents the antigen. Antigen presenting cells in the secondary lymphoid organs are specialized to provide this co-stimulation, but your everyday cells out in the tissues are not. To take advantage of this fact, T cells are programmed so that when they recognize their cognate antigen, but do not receive adequate co-stimulation, they are anergized or killed. Thus, even if cells in the tissues happen to express enough MHC-self peptide complexes to adequately crosslink the receptors on "lawbreaking" T cells, they generally don't express the co-stimulatory molecules required to rescue these T cells from death or anergy. Finally, even in the rare event that T cells are activated by cells in the tissues, these T cells usually die because they are chronically stimulated by the ever-present self antigens.

The picture you should have is that none of the mechanisms for tolerizing T cells is foolproof – they all are a little "leaky." However, because there are multiple layers of tolerance-inducing mechanisms to catch potentially self-reactive T cells, the whole system works very well, and relatively few humans suffer from serious autoimmune disease.

Tolerance induction in B cells is also multilayered. Unlike T cells, which have a separate organ, the thymus, in which central tolerance is induced, B cells with receptors that recognize relatively abundant self antigens are eliminated where they are born – in the bone marrow. Virgin B cells mainly traffic through the blood, lymph, and secondary lymphoid organs, where they are exposed to the same abundant self antigens that they "viewed" in the bone marrow. Naive B cells that wander out of this traffic pattern usually don't encounter sufficient self antigen in a form that can crosslink their BCRs. In addition, virgin B cells whose receptors are crosslinked by self antigen in tissues usually don't receive the co-stimulatory signals required for activation – and crosslinking without co-stimulation can anergize or kill B cells. Finally, if B cells are chronically re-stimulated (e.g., by self antigens out in the tissues), they eventually die by apoptosis, adding yet another layer of protection against self-reactivity.

IMMUNOPATHOLOGY

So far, we have focused on the "good" that the immune system does in protecting us from infection. Occasionally, however, the immune system "goes wrong" – sometimes with devastating consequences. In this lecture we will examine four categories of diseases in which the immune system plays a major role in producing the damaging effects (the pathology) of the disease. First, we will discuss examples of diseases in which the normal functioning of the immune system results in pathological consequences. Next, we will examine diseases that result when the systems that usually control the immune response don't function properly. Then we will discuss autoimmune diseases caused by a breakdown in the mechanisms that nor-

mally ensure tolerance of self. Finally, we will focus on diseases that stem from immunodeficiencies, both genetic and acquired.

PATHOLOGICAL CONDITIONS CAUSED BY A NORMAL IMMUNE RESPONSE

Tuberculosis is an excellent example of a disease whose pathological consequences are the result of normal immune system function. Tuberculosis is usually contracted by inhaling microdroplets containing the TB bacterium (*Mycobacterium tuberculosis*) that are generated by the cough of an infected individual. When these bacteria are taken into the lungs, they are confronted by macrophages that are stationed there to intercept invaders that enter via the respiratory tract.

From Lecture 1, you remember that a macrophage first engulfs an invader in a pouch (vesicle) called a phagosome. This vesicle is then taken inside the macrophage where it fuses with another vesicle called a lysosome, which contains powerful chemicals that can destroy the bacterium.

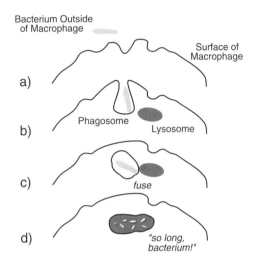

Unfortunately, in the case of the tuberculosis bacterium, the macrophage bites off more than it can chew, because the TB bacterium is able to modify the surface of the phagosome so that it does not fuse with the lysosome. Within the phagosome, the bacterium is safe, and it has easy access to all the nutrients it needs to grow and multiply. Eventually, many newly minted TB bacteria burst out of the macrophage, killing it. These bacteria then go on to infect other macrophages in the area. As a macrophage dies by necrosis, the contents of its lysosomes are released into the tissues of the lung. This causes tissue damage and initiates an inflammatory reaction that recruits other immune system cells to the battle site, causing even more tissue damage.

The struggle between macrophages and TB bacteria results in the production of battle cytokines that can hyperactivate macrophages in the lung. Once hyperactivated, macrophages can better deal with TB bacteria because the killing power of their weapons increases. However, some of the chemicals given off by hyperactivated macrophages also cause additional damage to the tissues of the lung.

Activated macrophages and the cells they recruit sometimes win this battle and eliminate the invading bacteria. In other cases, it's a fight to a draw, and a state of chronic inflammation results in which the bacteria are kept in check, but macrophages continue to be killed, and the lungs continue to be damaged by the inflammatory reaction. So in a TB infection, the pathology of the disease results from macrophages doing exactly what they are supposed to do – engulf invaders and summon additional immune system cells to help fight the battle.

Sepsis is another disease that is due to the immune system doing all the right things. Sepsis is a rather generic term that describes the symptoms that can result from a systemic infection. Such an infection is usually caused by bacteria that enter the blood when the physical barriers which are our first line of defense are breached. For sepsis to occur in a healthy individual, a large number of bacteria usually must be introduced. This could occur, for example, as a result of bacterial escape from an abscess or other formerly localized infection. In patients with a suppressed immune system (e.g., during chemotherapy for cancer), much smaller quantities of bacteria are required.

Although both Gram-negative and Gram-positive bacteria can cause sepsis, the classic culprits are Gram-negative bacteria like *E. coli* that have LPS (lipopolysaccharide) as a component of their cell walls, and which also shed this molecule into their surroundings. As we discussed in Lecture 2, LPS is a potent danger signal that can activate macrophages and NK cells. These two cells then work together in a positive feedback loop that increases their activation states and upregulates the production of cytokines which recruit neutrophils and additional macrophages and NK cells from the blood.

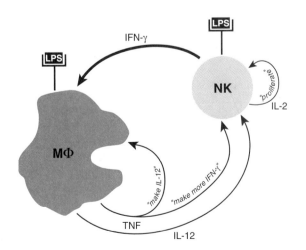

Under normal conditions, the function of this positive feedback loop is to amplify the immune response so that the innate system can respond quickly and strongly to a <u>localized</u> infection. However, in a "full-body" infection, in which bacteria carried by the blood enter tissues everywhere, this amplified response can get out of hand. TNF secreted by activated macrophages can cause blood vessels to become "leaky," so that fluid escapes from the vessels into the surrounding tissues. In extreme cases, the decrease in blood volume due to system-wide leakage can cause a drop in blood pressure that results in shock (septic shock) and heart failure. So sepsis and septic shock can result when the positive feedback loops that normally allow the innate immune system to react strongly and quickly to an invasion cause an overreaction to a system-wide infection.

DISEASES CAUSED BY DEFECTS IN IMMUNE REGULATION

Roughly a quarter of the U.S. population suffers from allergies to common environmental antigens (allergens) that are either inhaled or ingested. The immune systems of non-allergic individuals respond weakly to these allergens, and produce mainly low levels of IgG antibodies. In striking contrast, allergic individuals (called "atopic" individuals) produce large quantities of IgE antibodies. Indeed, the concentration of IgE antibodies in the blood of atopic individuals can be 1,000- to 10,000-fold higher than in the blood of non-atopic people! It is the overproduction of IgE antibodies in response to otherwise innocuous environmental antigens that causes allergies.

In Lecture 3, we discussed the interaction of IgE antibodies with white blood cells called mast cells. Since mast cell degranulation is a central event in many allergic reactions, let's take a moment to review this concept. When atopic individuals are first exposed to an allergen (e.g., pollen) they produce large amounts of IgE antibodies which recognize that allergen. Mast cells have receptors on their surfaces that can bind to the Fc region of IgE antibodies, so that after the initial exposure, mast cells will have large numbers of these allergen-specific IgE molecules attached to their surfaces. Allergens are small proteins with a repeating structure to which many IgE antibodies can bind close together. So on a second or subsequent exposure, the allergen can crosslink the IgE molecules on the mast cell surface, dragging the Fc receptors together. This clustering of Fc receptors signals mast cells to "degranulate" – to release the granules, which normally are stored safely inside the mast cells, into the tissues in which they reside. Mast cell granules contain histamine and other powerful chemicals and enzymes that can cause the symptoms with which atopic individuals are intimately familiar.

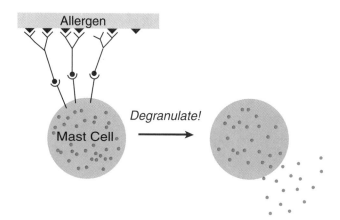

Interestingly, although IgE antibodies only live for about a day in the blood, once they are attached to mast cells they have a half life of several weeks. This means that mast cells can stay "armed" and ready to degranulate for an extended period after exposure to an allergen.

Allergic reactions generally have two phases: immediate and delayed. The immediate reaction to an allergen is the work of mast cells, which are stationed out in the tissues, and basophils, another granule-containing white blood cell, which can be recruited from the blood by signals given off by mast cells responding to an allergen. Like mast cells, basophils have receptors for IgE antibodies, and crosslinking of these receptors can lead to basophil degranulation. However, unlike mast cells, which are very long-lived in the tissues, basophils only live for a few days.

Although mast cells and basophils are responsible for the immediate reaction to an allergen, a third granule-containing white blood cell, the eosinophil, is the prominent player in chronic allergic reactions (e.g., in asthma). Before an "attack" by an allergen, there are relatively few eosinophils present in the tissues or circulating in the blood. However, once an allergic reaction has begun, helper T cells secrete cytokines, such as IL-5, that can recruit many more eosinophils from the bone marrow. These eosinophils can then add their "weight" to the allergic reaction. Because eosinophils must be mobilized from the marrow, their contribution is delayed relative to that of mast cells and basophils, which can respond almost immediately.

Of course, mast cells, basophils, and eosinophils were not invented by Mother Nature just to annoy allergic people. These cells, with their ability to degranulate "on command," provide a defense against parasites (e.g., worms) that are too large to be phagocytosed by professional phagocytes.

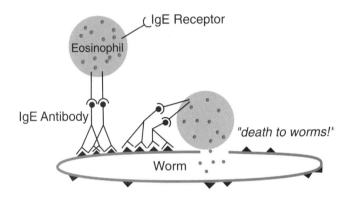

You may have noticed a parallel between the mast cell/basophil collaboration during a parasitic (or allergen) attack and the macrophage/neutrophil collaboration that takes place during a bacterial infection. In both cases, a long-lived "sentinel" cell, which resides in the tissues, is activated in response to an invader, and then summons short-lived "hired guns" from the blood to help with the battle.

It is clear that IgE antibodies are the bad guys in allergic reactions, but what determines whether a person will make IgE or IgG antibodies in response to an allergen? You remember from Lecture 5 that helper T cells can be influenced by the environment in which they are re-stimulated to secrete various cytokines, and that their cytokine profiles can be polarized toward the production of a Th1 or Th2 subset of cytokines.

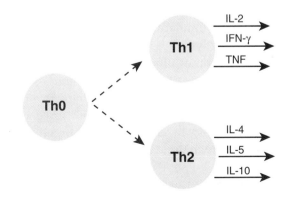

In turn, B cells undergoing class switching are influenced to switch to production of IgA, IgG, or IgE antibodies, depending on the cytokines produced by helper T cells in the germinal centers where class switching takes place. For example, a germinal center that is populated with Th1 cells usually will produce B cells that make IgG antibodies, because Th1 cells secrete IFN-γ, which drives the IgG class switch. In contrast, B cells tend to change to IgE production if they class switch in germinal centers that contain Th2 cells, which secrete IL-4 and IL-5. So the decision to produce either IgG or IgE antibodies in response to an allergen will depend mainly on the type of helper T cells present in the secondary lymphoid organs that happen to intercept the allergen. Indeed, helper T cells from allergic individuals show a much stronger bias toward the Th2 type than do Th cells from non-atopic people.

Okay, so atopic individuals produce IgE antibodies because their allergen-specific helper T cells tend to be of the Th2 type. But how do they get that way? The answer to this question is not known for certain, but many immunologists believe that a bias toward either Th1- or Th2-type helper T cells is usually established early in childhood, and in some cases, even before birth. Here's how this is thought to work.

A fetus inherits roughly half its genetic material from its mother and half from its father, and as a result, the fetus is really a "transplant" that expresses many paternal antigens to which the mother's immune system is not tolerant. Since the placenta is the interface between the mother and the fetus, measures must be taken to avoid having maternal CTLs and NK cells attack the placenta because it expresses these paternal antigens. The Th1 subset of helper cells secretes TNF, which helps activate NK cells, and IL-2, which causes NK cells and CTLs to proliferate. So it would be advantageous for the survival of the fetus to bias maternal Th cells away from the Th1 cytokine profile. Indeed, cells of the placenta produce relatively large amounts of IL-4 and IL-10 – cytokines that influence maternal helper T cells to become Th2 cells. However, these same placental cytokines also have a strong influence on <u>fetal</u> helper T cells. As a result, most humans are born with helper T cells that are strongly biased toward making Th2 cytokines.

Obviously, this bias does not last a lifetime, and eventually most people end up with a more balanced population of Th1 and Th2 cells. One event that probably helps establish this balance is infection at an early age with microbes (e.g., viruses or bacteria) that normally elicit a Th1 response. Indeed, it is suspected that early microbial infections may also be important in "re-programming" the immune response so that a Th1 response to allergens results. Immunologists hypothesize that if a microbial infection strongly "deviates" the immune response of a young child toward a Th1 type at the same time that the child encounters an allergen (say, a dust mite protein), the Th response to that allergen will also be deviated toward the Th1 type. Once this deviation takes place, feedback mechanisms will tend to lock in the Th1 response, and memory T cells will be generated that remember not only the allergen, but also their Th1 response to it. Once a large number of biased memory cells is built up, it is difficult to reverse this bias, so early exposure to infectious diseases may be critical in establishing a normal response to environmental allergens.

This concept of "immune deviation" is consistent with the increased incidence of allergies and the corresponding decreased incidence of microbial infections (e.g., tuberculosis) seen in developed countries, and is sometimes referred to as the "hygiene hypothesis." The existence of a window of opportunity during which a child is susceptible to immune deviation could also explain the finding that children born at certain times of the year are more likely to develop seasonal allergies.

In addition to environmental factors (e.g., early exposure to infectious diseases), heredity clearly plays a large part in susceptibility to allergies. For example, if one identical twin suffers from allergies, the probability is about 50% that the second twin will also be atopic. Immunologists have noticed that people who are allergic to certain allergens are more likely to have inherited particular class II MHC genes than are non-atopic people, suggesting that these MHC molecules may be especially efficient at presenting allergens. In addition, some atopic individuals produce mutant forms of the IgE receptor. It is hypothesized that these mutant receptors send an unusually strong signal when crosslinked, resulting in secretion of abnormally high levels of IL-4 by mast cells, and favoring the production of IgE antibodies. Mutations have even been detected in the regulatory (promoter) region of the IL-4 gene of some atopic individuals, and these mutations might increase the amount of IL-4 produced. Unfortunately, genes that confer susceptibility to allergies have been difficult to identify, because there seem to be many of them, and because they differ from atopic individual to atopic individual.

The best current synthesis of this information is that the immunological basis for allergies is a defect in immune regulation in which allergen-specific helper T cells are strongly polarized toward the Th2 cytokine profile, resulting in the production of allergen-specific IgE antibodies. The genes a person inherits can make him or her more or less susceptible to allergies, and exposure to environmental factors such as microbial infections may influence whether susceptible individuals become atopic.

AUTOIMMUNE DISEASE

Rather than expend a huge amount of biological "energy" on a foolproof system in which every B and T cell is carefully checked for tolerance to self, Mother Nature evolved a multilayered system in which each layer includes mechanisms that should weed out most self-reactive cells, with lower layers catching cells that slip through tolerance induction in the layers above. This strategy works very well, but occasionally "mistakes are made," and the system breaks down. Autoimmune disease results when a breakdown in the mechanisms meant to preserve tolerance of self is severe enough to cause a pathological condition. Unfortunately, roughly 5% of Americans suffers from some form of autoimmune disease.

Autoimmune disorders can result from genetic defects. For example, most autoimmune diseases are chronic disorders that involve repeated stimulation of self-reactive lymphocytes. In normal people, this is controlled by activation-induced cell death in which chronically stimulated T cells are eliminated when Fas proteins on their surfaces are ligated. Humans with genetic defects in either Fas or Fas ligand proteins lack this layer of tolerance protection, and their T cells refuse to die when chronically stimulated by self antigens. The resulting diseases, autoimmune lymphoproliferative syndrome and Canale-Smith syndrome, have as their pathologic consequences massive swelling of lymph nodes, production of antibodies that recognize self antigens, and the accumulation of large numbers of T cells in the secondary lymphoid organs.

Although some autoimmune disorders are due to genetic defects, the majority of autoimmune diseases occur when the layers of tolerance inducing mechanisms fail to eliminate self-reactive cells in genetically normal individuals. In fact, you could argue that the potential for autoimmune disease is the price we must pay for having T and B cell receptors which are so diverse that they can recognize essentially any invader.

The latest thinking is that for autoimmunity to occur, at least three conditions must be met. First, an individual must express MHC molecules that can efficiently present a peptide derived from the target self antigen. This means that the MHC molecules you inherit can play a major role in determining susceptibility to autoimmune disease. For example, only about 0.2% of the U.S. population suffers from juvenile diabetes, yet for Caucasian Americans who inherit two particular types of class II MHC genes, the probability of contracting this autoimmune disease is increased about twenty-fold.

The second requirement for autoimmunity is that the afflicted person must produce T and in some cases B cells that have receptors which recognize a self antigen. Because TCRs and BCRs are made by a mix and match strategy, the repertoire of receptors that one individual expresses will be different from that of every other individual, and will change with time as lymphocytes die and are replaced. Even the collections of TCRs and BCRs expressed by identical twins will be different. Therefore, it is largely by chance that a person will produce lymphocytes whose receptors recognize a particular self antigen.

So, for autoimmune disease to occur, a person must have MHC molecules that can present self antigens, and T cells with receptors that can recognize these presented antigens – but this is not enough. In addition, there must be environmental factors that lead to the breakdown of the normal tolerance mechanisms that are designed to eliminate self-reactive lymphocytes. For years, physicians have noticed that autoimmune diseases frequently follow bacterial or viral infections, and immunologists now believe that microbial attack may be one of the key environmental factors that triggers autoimmune disease. Now clearly, a viral or bacterial infection cannot be the whole story, because for most people these infections do not result in autoimmunity. However, in conjunction with a genetic predisposition (e.g., type of MHC molecules inherited) and lymphocytes with potentially self-reactive receptors, a microbial infection may be the "last straw" that leads to autoimmune disease.

MOLECULAR MIMICRY

Immunologists' current favorite hypothesis to explain why infections might lead to a breakdown in self tolerance is called "molecular mimicry." Here's how this is thought to work.

Lymphocytes have BCRs or TCRs that recognize their cognate antigen. It turns out, however, that this is almost never a single antigen. Just as one MHC molecule can present a large number of peptides that have the same general characteristics (length, binding motif, etc.), a TCR or a BCR usually can recognize ("cross react" with) several different antigens. Generally, a TCR or BCR will have a high affinity for one or a few of these cognate antigens, and relatively lower affinities for the others.

During a microbial invasion, B or T cells whose receptors recognize microbial antigens will be activated. The molecular mimicry hypothesis holds that sometimes these receptors also recognize self antigens, and if they do, an autoimmune response to the self antigens can result. It is presumed that before the microbial infection, these potentially self-reactive lymphocytes had not been activated either because the affinities of their receptors for self antigens were too low to trigger activation, or because the restricted traffic patterns of virgin lymphocytes never brought them into contact with self antigens under conditions that would allow activation. However, once activated in response to a cross-reacting microbial antigen, these self-reactive lymphocytes can now do real damage. For example, it is believed that rheumatic heart disease, which is a possible complication of a streptococcal throat infection, results when the receptors on helper T cells that recognize streptococcal antigens cross react with proteins present on the tissues that make up the mitral valve of the heart. These cross-reactive Th cells appear to direct an inflammatory response that can severely damage the heart valve.

Animal models of human autoimmune diseases have been very useful for understanding which immune system players are involved, which self antigens are targets of the immune reaction, and which microbial antigens might be involved in the molecular mimicry that may trigger disease. Typically, these models involve animals that have been bred to be exquisitely susceptible to autoimmune disease, or animals whose genes have been altered to make them susceptible. One lesson learned from animal models and from humans is that TCRs which recognize self antigens can cross react with multiple environmental antigens. Consequently, although viral or bacterial infections may supply the environmental trigger for some autoimmune diseases, it appears unlikely that any single microbe is responsible for any one autoimmune disease.

INFLAMMATION AND AUTOIMMUNE DISEASE

Although molecular mimicry may be responsible for activating lymphocytes that previously had been "ignorant" of self antigens, there must be more to the story. After all, when self-reactive T cells activated by a microbial mimic reach the tissues, they are in a precarious situation. To avoid apoptotic death by "neglect," they must be continuously re-stimulated, and if they encounter self antigens in an environment that does not provide adequate co-stimulation, they will be anergized or deleted.

As you remember, the innate system usually gives "permission" for the adaptive system to function. Part of this permission involves the activation of antigen presenting cells by inflammatory cytokines such as IFN-γ and TNF that are secreted by cells of the innate system. Once activated, APCs (e.g., macrophages) will express the MHC and co-stimulatory molecules that are required to re-stimulate T cells which have entered the tissues. What this means is that when lymphocytes venture out into the tissues to join a battle that the innate system is already fighting, re-stimulation is not a problem. However, for a T cell that recognizes a self antigen which the innate system does not see as dangerous, the tissues can be a very inhospitable place – because the self-reactive lymphocyte usually will not receive the co-stimulation necessary for its survival.

The bottom line is that it is not enough for a microbe to activate self-reactive T cells by mimicry. There must also be an inflammatory reaction going on in the same tissues that express the self antigen. Otherwise it is unlikely that self-reactive lymphocytes would exit the blood into these tissues, and if they did, that they would survive. This requirement for inflammation probably explains why bacterial infections (e.g., strep throat) rarely lead to autoimmune disease (e.g., rheumatic heart disease).

So the scenario most immunologists favor for the initiation of autoimmune disease is this: An individual who is genetically susceptible is attacked by a microbe that activates T cells whose receptors just happen to cross react with a self antigen. Simultaneously, an inflammatory reaction takes place in the tissues where the self antigen is expressed. This inflammation could be caused either by the mimicking microbe itself, or by another, unrelated infection or trauma. As a result of this inflammatory reaction, APCs are activated that can re-stimulate self-reactive T cells. In addition, cytokines generated by the inflammatory response can upregulate class I MHC expression on normal cells in the tissues, making these cells better targets for destruction by self-reactive CTLs.

EXAMPLES OF AUTOIMMUNE DISEASE

Autoimmune diseases are usually divided into two groups: organ-specific and multi-system diseases. Let's look at examples of both types, paying special attention to the self antigens against which the autoimmune response is thought to be directed, and to the environmental antigens that may be involved in molecular mimicry.

One important example of an organ-specific autoimmune disease is insulin-dependent diabetes mellitus. In this disease, the targets of autoimmune attack are the insulin-producing "β cells" of the pancreas. Although antibodies produced by self-reactive B cells may participate in the chronic inflammation that contributes to the pathology of this disease, it is currently believed that the initial attack on the β cells is mediated by CTLs.

Clearly, there are genetic factors that help determine susceptibility to diabetes, since the probability that both identical twins will have this autoimmune disease is about 50% if one of them has it. Thus far, no strong candidates have emerged for environmental factors that might trigger the initial attack on β cells. However, many immunologists believe that diabetes results, at least in part, when "regulatory T cells," which should keep self-reactive CTLs under control, don't function properly. Unfortunately, it remains to be discovered exactly what "under control" means in this situation, and how these regulatory T cells accomplish this feat.

In diabetes, destruction of insulin-producing cells in the pancreas usually begins months or even years before the first symptoms of diabetes appear, so this disease is sometimes referred to as a "silent killer." Fortunately, antibodies that bind to β cell antigens are produced very early in the disease. As a result, relatives of diabetic patients can be tested to determine whether they are making these self-reactive antibodies and therefore might be in the early stages of diabetes.

Myasthenia gravis is an autoimmune disease that results when self-reactive antibodies bind to the receptor for an important neurotransmitter, acetylcholine. When the message that is normally carried by acetylcholine from nerve to muscle is not received (because the antibodies interfere with its reception), muscle weakness and paralysis can result. Immunologists have noticed that a region of one of the poliovirus proteins is similar in amino acid sequence to part of the acetylcholine receptor, so it is possible that a polio infection might provide one mimic which could activate lymphocytes whose receptors cross react with the acetylcholine receptor.

Multiple sclerosis is an inflammatory disease of the central nervous system that is thought to be initiated by self-reactive T cells. In multiple sclerosis, chronic inflammation destroys the myelin sheaths that are required for nerve cells in the brain to transmit electrical signals efficiently, causing defects in sensory inputs (e.g., vision) and paralysis. Macrophages recruited by cytokines secreted by T cells are thought to play a major role in causing this inflammation. At first there was a question as to how T cells could get into the brain to initiate this disease, but eventually it was discovered that activated T cells (but not virgin T cells) can cross the blood-brain barrier. The presumed target of these T cells is a major component of the myelin sheath: myelin basic protein. T cells isolated from multiple sclerosis patients can recognize a peptide derived from myelin basic protein as well as peptides derived from proteins encoded by both herpes simplex virus and Epstein-Barr virus (the virus that causes mononucleosis). So a possible scenario is that when genetically susceptible individuals are infected with herpes virus or Epstein-Barr virus, they produce T cells that recognize proteins from these viruses. Some of these activated T cells may have receptors that cross react with myelin basic protein, and once these T cells cross the blood-brain barrier, they can lead the attack on the myelin sheaths, causing the symptoms of multiple sclerosis.

Of course, very few people who have Epstein-Barr or herpes infections get multiple sclerosis, so exposure to microbial mimics is not the whole story. Indeed, as is true of most autoimmune diseases, multiple sclerosis has a strong genetic component: It is about ten times more probable that identical twins will share this disease than it is for non-identical twins to both be afflicted. In addition, it is about twenty times more likely that the non-identical twin of someone with multiple sclerosis will also have the disease than it is for a person in the general population. Moreover, there are certain "resistant" groups (e.g., Hispanic, Asian, Native American) who have relatively low rates of multiple sclerosis, presumably because of their particular genetic makeup.

Pemphigus vulgaris is an autoimmune disease in which antibodies to a self protein (desmoglein I) on the surface of skin cells disrupt the adhesion between these cells, resulting in the formation of blisters on the skin. In fact, antibodies obtained from pemphigus patients can cause symptoms of the disease when injected into animals. Interestingly, a gene encoding one particular type of class II MHC molecule has so far only been found in patients with pemphigus, suggesting that the types of MHC molecules a person inherits can play a major role in determining susceptibility to this disease.

Rheumatoid arthritis is a systemic autoimmune disease that is characterized by chronic inflammation of the joints. One of the presumed targets of this autoimmune reaction is a certain cartilage protein, and T cells from arthritic patients can recognize both the cartilage protein and a protein encoded by the bacterium that causes tuberculosis. In this regard, it is interesting that mice injected with *Mycobacterium tuberculosis* suffer from inflammation of the joints, suggesting, <u>but not proving</u>, that a mycobacterial infection may trigger rheumatoid arthritis in some patients.

IgM antibodies that can bind to the tails of IgG antibodies are found in the joints of individuals with rheumatoid arthritis. These antibodies can form IgM-IgG antibody complexes which can activate macrophages that have entered the joints, increasing the inflammatory reaction. Indeed, the inflammation associated with rheumatoid arthritis is caused mainly by tumor necrosis factor (TNF) produced by macrophages that infiltrate the joints under the direction of self-reactive helper T cells. To treat arthritis, two drugs are currently being used that "soak up" TNF. One is an antibody that binds to TNF and prevents it from working, and the other is a fake receptor for TNF. Both of these "blockade" strategies are very effective in decreasing the severity of the symptoms experienced by patients with rheumatoid arthritis.

Finally, lupus erythematosus is a systemic autoimmune disease that affects about 250,000 people in the U.S., roughly 90% of whom are women. This disease can have multiple manifestations, including a red rash on the forehead and cheeks (giving the "red wolf" appearance for which the disease was named), inflammation of the lungs, arthritis, kidney damage, hair loss, paralysis, and convulsions. Lupus is caused by a breakdown in both B and T cell tolerance that results in the production of a diverse collection of IgG antibodies which recognize a wide range of self antigens including DNA,

DNA-protein complexes, and RNA-protein complexes. In lupus, the diversity of self antibodies produced is thought to be reflected in the diversity of the disease symptoms experienced by individual patients. These autoantibodies can form self antigen-antibody complexes which may "clog" organs in the body that contain "filters" (e.g., kidneys, joints, and the brain), causing chronic inflammation.

Non-identical twins have about a 2% probability of both having lupus, whereas with identical twins, this probability increases about ten-fold. This indicates a strong genetic component to the disease, and multiple MHC and non-MHC genes have been identified, each of which seems to slightly increase the probability that a person will contract lupus. Although no specific microbial infection has been associated with the initiation of this autoimmune disease, mice that lack functional genes for Fas or Fas ligand exhibit lupus-like symptoms. This has led immunologists to speculate that lupus may involve a defect in activation-induced cell death, in which lymphocytes that should die due to chronic stimulation survive to cause the disease.

ANTIGEN SPREADING

One of the reasons it has been so difficult for immunologists to identify environmental factors (e.g., specific microbes) that trigger autoimmune disease is the phenomenon of "antigen spreading." When T or B cells are isolated from patients with autoimmune disease, collectively these lymphocytes usually recognize several, and in some cases many, self antigens. What seems to be happening is that although autoimmunity may originally involve T or B cells that recognize a single "initiating" self antigen, with time other lymphocytes that recognize additional self antigens also are activated.

For example, it is suspected that lupus is initiated by T and B cells that recognize DNA coated with proteins (as DNA normally is in human cells) which have been released from cells damaged by infection or trauma. Once started, the autoimmune response results in the recruitment of macrophages and additional immune system cells. These "recruits" amplify the inflammatory response at the site by expressing cytokines such as IFN-γ and TNF that increase the efficiency of antigen presentation by macrophages and dendritic cells. The result is that other self antigens that have been released from damaged tissues, and which

formerly were poorly presented due to inadequate MHC expression or inadequate co-stimulation, now can be presented efficiently enough to activate T cells that had previously ignored their existence. Consequently, the targets of self-reacting T cells "spread" from the initiating self antigen to other self antigens that originally were "quiet" enough to be ignored.

DISEASES DUE TO IMMUNODEFICIENCIES

Serious disease may result when our immune systems do not operate at full strength. Some of these immunodeficiencies are caused by genetic defects that disable parts of the immune network. Others are "acquired" as the consequence of malnutrition, deliberate immunosuppression (e.g., during organ transplantation or chemotherapy for cancer), or disease (e.g., AIDS).

GENETIC DEFECTS LEADING TO IMMUNODEFICIENCY

A genetic defect in which a single gene is mutated can lead to immune system weakness. For example, individuals who are born with non-functional CD40 or CD40L proteins are unable to mount a T cell-dependent antibody response, because T cells either cannot deliver or B cells cannot receive the all-important, co-stimulatory signal. The result of the CD40-CD40L defect is that B cells secrete mainly IgM antibodies that have not affinity matured, because both class switching and somatic hypermutation require co-stimulation by CD40L.

Other genetic deficiencies affect the formation of the thymus. In one such deficiency, DiGeorge syndrome, essentially all thymic tissue is missing, and people with this disorder are susceptible to life-threatening infections because they lack functional T cells.

Genetic defects can also knock out both T and B cells. This group of diseases is called severe combined immunodeficiency syndrome (SCIDS) – where the "combined" label indicates that neither T nor B cells function properly. It was because of this disease that the famous "bubble boy" had to be kept isolated in a pathogen-free environment. Although a number of different mutations can result in SCIDS, the best-studied mutation causes a defect in a protein that initiates the gene splicing required to produce mature B and T cell receptors. Without their receptors, T and B cells are blind to the world around them and are totally useless.

Immunodeficiencies also can result from genetic defects in the innate immune system. For example, people who are born with defects in important complement proteins (e.g., C3) have lymph nodes with an abnormal architecture (no germinal centers) and B cells that produce mainly IgM antibodies.

Given the large number of different proteins that are involved in making the innate and adaptive immune systems work effectively, it's pretty amazing that mutations leading to immunodeficiency are quite rare. In fact, inherited immunodeficiencies afflict only about one in 10,000 newborns. It is likely, however, that many other cases of genetic immunodeficiency go undetected because our "redundant" immune system has evolved to provide "backups" when elements of the main system are disabled.

AIDS

Although genetic immunodeficiencies are relatively rare, millions of people suffer from immunodeficiencies that are acquired. A large group of immunodeficient humans acquired their deficiency when they were infected with the AIDS virus – a virus that currently infects over forty million people worldwide. The AIDS symptoms that originally alerted physicians that they were dealing with a disease that had immunodeficiency as its basis was the high incidence of infections (e.g., *Pneumocystis carinii* pneumonia) or cancers (e.g., Kaposi's sarcoma) that were usually only seen in immunosuppressed individuals. Soon, the virus that caused this immunodeficiency was isolated and named the human immunodeficiency virus number one (HIV-1).

An HIV-1 infection begins very much like other viral infections. Viruses in the initial inoculum enter human cells, and use these cells' biosynthetic machinery to make many more copies of themselves. These newly made viruses then burst out of the cell, and go on to infect other cells. So in the early stages of infection, the virus multiplies relatively unchecked while the innate system gives it its best shot, and the adaptive system is being mobilized. After a week or so, the adaptive system starts to kick in, and virus-specific B cells, helper T cells, and CTLs are activated, proliferate, and begin to do their thing. During this early, "acute" phase

of a viral infection, there is a dramatic rise in the number of viruses in the body (viral load) as the virus multiplies in infected cells. This is followed by a marked decrease in the viral load as virus-specific CTLs and antibodies go to work.

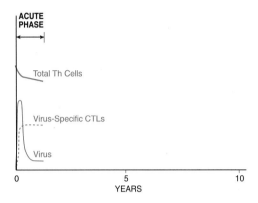

With many types of virus (e.g., smallpox), the end result of the acute phase of a viral infection is "sterilization": All the invading viruses are destroyed, and memory B and T cells are produced to protect against a subsequent infection by the same virus. There is some evidence that for a few, very lucky individuals, an HIV-1 infection may also end in sterilization. However, for the vast majority, infection with HIV-1 leads next to a "chronic" phase that can last for ten or more years. During this phase, a fierce struggle goes on between the immune system and the AIDS virus – a struggle that, unfortunately, the virus always seems to win.

During the chronic phase of infection, viral loads decrease to low levels compared with those reached during the height of the acute phase, and the number of virus-specific CTLs and Th cells remains high – a sign that the immune system is still trying hard to defeat the virus.

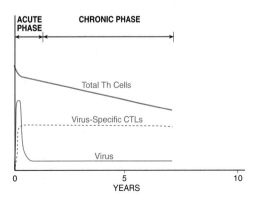

However, as the chronic phase progresses, the total number of Th cells slowly decreases, because these cells are killed as a consequence of the viral infection. Eventually there are not enough Th cells left to provide the help needed by the virus-specific CTLs. When this happens, the number of CTLs also begins to decline, and the viral load increases – because there are too few CTLs left to cope with newly-infected cells.

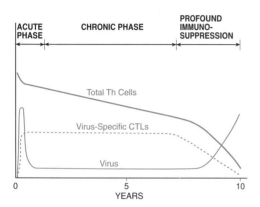

In the end, the immune defenses are overwhelmed, and the resulting profound state of immunosuppression leaves the patient open to unchecked infections by pathogens that would normally not be the slightest problem for a person with an intact immune system. Sadly, these "opportunistic" infections can be lethal to an AIDS patient whose immune system has been destroyed.

Why is HIV-1 able to defeat an immune system that is so successful in protecting us from most other pathogens? There are two parts to this answer. The first has to do with the nature of the virus itself. All viruses are basically pieces of genetic information (either DNA or RNA) with a protective coat. For the AIDS virus, this genetic information is in the form of RNA, which after the virus enters its target cell, is copied by a viral enzyme called reverse transcriptase to make a piece of complementary ("copy") DNA (cDNA). Next, the DNA of the cell is cut by another enzyme carried by the virus, and the viral cDNA is inserted into the gap in the cellular DNA. Now comes the nasty part. Once the viral DNA has been inserted into cellular DNA, it can just sit there, and while the virus is in this "latent" state, the infected cell cannot be detected by CTLs. Sometime later, in response to signals that are not fully understood, the latent virus can "reactivate," more copies of the virus can be produced, and these newly minted viruses can then infect other cells.

So the ability to establish a latent infection that cannot be detected by CTLs is one property of HIV-1 that makes it such a problem. But it gets worse. The reverse transcriptase enzyme used to copy the viral RNA is very error-prone: It makes about one error (mutation) each time it copies a piece of viral RNA into cDNA. What this means is that the new viruses produced in an infected cell usually are different from the virus that originally infected that cell. These mutations can have three results. First, the mutations may not change the viral structure or function at all. Second, the mutations may actually kill the virus, because they disturb some essential function (e.g., the mutation might change the reverse transcriptase so that it no longer can copy viral RNA). Finally (and this is the scary part), the mutations may help the virus adapt to its environment, so that it can become even more damaging.

For example, the virus might mutate so that a viral peptide that formerly was targeted by a CTL no longer can be recognized, or no longer can be presented by the MHC molecule that the CTL was trained to focus on. When such mutations occur, that CTL will be useless against cells infected with the mutant virus, and new CTLs that recognize another viral peptide will have to be activated. Meanwhile, the virus that has escaped from surveillance by the obsolete CTLs is replicating like crazy, and every time it infects a new cell, it mutates again. Consequently, the mutation rate of the AIDS virus is so high that it can effectively stay one step ahead of CTLs or antibodies directed against it.

So two of the properties of HIV-1 that make it especially deadly are its ability to establish an undetectable, latent infection, and its high mutation rate. But that's only half the story. The other part has to do with the cells HIV-1 infects. This virus specifically targets cells of the immune system: helper T cells, macrophages, and dendritic cells. The "docking" protein that HIV-1 binds to when it infects a cell is CD4, the co-receptor protein found in large numbers on the surfaces of helper T cells. This protein is also expressed on macrophages and dendritic cells, although they have fewer CD4 molecules on their surfaces. By attacking these cells, the AIDS virus either disrupts their function, kills the cells, or makes them targets for killing by CTLs that recognize them as being virus-infected. So the very cells that are needed to activate CTLs and to provide them with help are damaged or destroyed by the virus.

Even more insidiously, HIV-1 can turn the immune system against itself by using processes essential for immune function to spread and maintain the viral infection. For example, HIV-1 can attach to the surfaces of dendritic cells and be transported by these cells from the tissues, where there are relatively few CD4$^+$ cells, into the lymph nodes, where huge numbers of CD4$^+$ T cells are located. Not only are there lots of CD4$^+$ cells within easy reach in lymph nodes, but many of these cells are proliferating, making them ideal candidates for HIV-1 "factories." As far as HIV-1 is concerned, a lymph node is about as close to heaven as a virus can get.

AIDS viruses that have been opsonized either by antibodies or by complement are retained in lymph nodes by follicular dendritic cells. This display is intended to help activate B cells. However, CD4$^+$ T cells also pass through these forests of FDCs, and as they do, they can be infected by HIV-1 particles that are attached to the dendritic cell "trees." Because virus particles typically remain bound to follicular dendritic cells for months, lymph nodes actually become reservoirs of HIV-1. So by choosing to infect CD4$^+$ cells, HIV-1 takes advantage of the normal trafficking of immune system cells through lymph nodes and turns these "dating bars" into its own playground.

In summary, the pathological consequences of an HIV-1 infection are the result of the virus's ability to slowly destroy the immune system of the patient, leading to a state of profound immunosuppression that eventually results in death. The virus is able to do this because it can establish a latent, "stealth" infection, because it has a high mutation rate, and because it preferentially infects and disables the very immune system cells that would normally defend against it.

THOUGHT QUESTIONS

1. Describe the events that lead to the degranulation of mast cells during an allergic reaction.
2. Why do some people have allergies, whereas others do not?
3. What events are likely to be required to initiate an autoimmune reaction?
4. Describe what happens to a patient's immune system during the course of an HIV-1 infection.
5. Discuss the features of an HIV-1 infection that make it so difficult for the immune system to deal with.

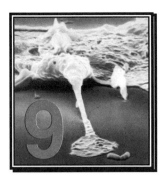

CANCER AND THE IMMUNE SYSTEM

In this, our last lecture, we're going to discuss how the immune system deals with cancer. Because some of you may not have had a cancer course, I think I'd better start by talking a bit about cancer cells. After all, it's important to know the enemy.

CANCER IS A CONTROL SYSTEM PROBLEM

Cancer arises when multiple control systems within a single cell are corrupted. These control systems are of two basic types: systems that promote cell growth (proliferation), and safeguard systems that protect against "irresponsible" cell growth. When controlled properly, cell proliferation is a good thing. After all, an adult human is made up of trillions of cells, so a lot of proliferation must take place between the time we are a single fertilized egg and the time we are full-grown. However, once a human reaches adulthood, most cell proliferation ceases. For example, when the cells in your kidney have proliferated to make that organ exactly the right size, the kidney cells stop growing. On the other hand, skin cells and cells that line our body cavities (e.g., our intestines) must proliferate almost continuously to replenish cells that are lost as these surfaces are eroded by normal wear and tear. All this cell proliferation, from cradle to grave, must be carefully controlled to insure that the right amount of proliferation takes place at the right places in the body and at the right times.

Usually, the growth-promoting systems within our cells work just fine. However, occasionally one of these systems may malfunction, and a cell may begin to proliferate inappropriately. When this happens, that cell has taken the first step toward becoming a cancer cell. Because the growth-promoting systems in cells are made up of proteins, malfunctions usually occur when a gene that specifies one of these proteins is mutated. A gene that, when mutated, can cause a cell to proliferate inappropriately is called a "proto-oncogene." And the mutated version of such a gene is called an "oncogene." The important point here is that uncontrolled cell growth can result when a normal cellular gene is mutated.

To protect against malfunctions in the control systems that promote cell proliferation, Mother Nature has equipped cells with "safeguard" systems. These safeguard systems are also made up of proteins, and they are of two general types: systems that help prevent mutations, and systems that deal with these mutations once they occur. For example, cells have a number of different "repair" systems that can fix damaged DNA, safeguarding against mutations. These DNA repair systems are especially important because mutations occur continually in the DNA of all our cells. In fact, it is estimated that, on average, each of our cells suffers about 25,000 mutational events every day. Fortunately, repair systems work nonstop, and if the DNA damage is relatively small, it can be immediately repaired as part of the "maintenance" repair program.

Sometimes, however, the maintenance repair systems may "miss" a mutation (e.g., if there are many mutations and the repair systems are overwhelmed). When this happens, a second type of safeguard system comes into play – one that monitors unrepaired mutations. If the mutations are not extensive, this safeguard system stops the cell from proliferating to give the repair systems more time to do their thing. However, if the genetic damage is severe, the safeguard system will trigger the cell to commit suicide, eliminating the possibility that it will become a cancer cell. One of the important components of this safeguard system is a protein called p53. Proteins like p53, which help safeguard against uncontrolled cell growth, are called "tumor suppressors," and the genes that encode them are called "anti-oncogenes" or "tumor suppressor genes." Clearly, p53 is part of an important safeguard system. Mutations in p53 have been detected in the majority of human tumors, and scientists have now created mice with mutant p53 genes. In contrast to normal mice, which rarely get cancer, mice that lack functional p53 proteins usually die of cancer before they are seven months old. So, if you are ever asked to give up one gene, don't pick p53!

The take-home lesson is that every normal cell has both proto-oncogenes and tumor suppressor genes. Where things get dangerous is when proto-oncogenes are mutated so that the cell proliferates inappropriately, and tumor suppressor genes are mutated so that the cell can't defend itself against proto-oncogenes "gone wrong." Indeed, cancer results when multiple control systems, both growth-promoting and safeguard, are corrupted within a single cell. It is estimated that between four and seven such mutations are required to produce most common cancers. This is the reason that cancer is a disease which generally strikes late in life: It usually takes a long time to accumulate the multiple mutations required to inappropriately activate growth-promoting systems and to disable safeguard systems.

Mutations that affect growth-promoting systems and safeguard systems can occur in any order. For example, one mutation that is especially insidious is a genetic alteration that disrupts one of the safeguard systems involved in repairing mutated DNA. When this happens, the mutation rate in a cell can soar, making it much more likely that the cell will accrue the multiple mutations required to turn it into a cancer cell. This type of "mutation-accelerating" defect is found in many (perhaps all) cancer cells. Indeed, one of the hallmarks of a cancer cell is a genetically unstable condition in which cellular genes are constantly mutating.

In addition to mutations in cellular genes that can corrupt growth-promoting and safeguard systems, some viruses produce proteins that can interfere with the proper functioning of these same systems in virus-infected cells. The net effect of such a viral infection is to decrease the total number of cellular genes that must be mutated to turn a normal cell into a cancer cell.

STAGES IN THE LIFE OF A CANCER CELL

Let's take a look at the changes that occur as a normal cell accumulates mutations and becomes a cancer cell. As you will see, there are many obstacles that a "wannabe" cancer cell must overcome.

First, a wannabe cancer cell must "learn" to proliferate inappropriately. Most of the time, this unnatural growth will be sensed by safeguard systems within the cell, and the cell will be instructed to die by apoptosis. This type of internal surveillance is probably sufficient to deal with most of the wannabes. Occasionally, however, when mutations occur in both proto-oncogenes and anti-oncogenes, human cells can begin to proliferate inappropriately. If you look carefully at your face, for example, you may see the result of inappropriate proliferation – what doctors call "benign growths." The older you get, the more of these you will notice, because they result from mutations that accumulate over time. An old guy like me has lots of them! What keeps these cells from making a huge growth on your face is that they haven't figured out how to overcome the next obstacle for wannabe cancer cells – the lack of a sufficient blood supply. All of our cells get their nourishment from the blood, and as a result, no living cell in your body is more than about a tenth of a millimeter from a blood vessel. So for a wannabe cancer cell to proliferate to form a mass of any size, growth-promoting systems within the cell must be activated which cause the cell to produce factors (angiogenic factors) that promote the growth of new blood vessels within the tumor.

Angiogenic factors can also be secreted by perfectly normal cells. For example, during embryonic development new blood vessels are required to supply nutrients to newly formed tissues and organs. In addition, angiogenic factors are made by normal cells in response to injury when new blood vessels are needed to replace those that have been damaged. So the systems required to produce angiogenic factors are present in normal cells – it's just that these growth-promoting systems generally are turned off.

Fortunately, most of the time the angiogenesis control systems operate normally, new blood vessels are not produced, and the growths on your face remain quite small. However, every once in a while, a wannabe cell may suffer additional mutations that result in the inappropriate secretion of angiogenic factors. If this happens, the new blood vessels that are produced make it possible for the wannabe cancer cells to acquire all the nourishment they need to continue to proliferate – and then the growth can become large. I think most of us have an "Old Uncle Harry" who has a big growth like this on his face. Fortunately, it is usually still benign, and if it gets too big (or too obnoxious!), a dermatologist can remove it. The growth is considered benign because it grows slowly, and because the wannabe cancer cells that make up the growth have not learned the deadliest trick of all – how to metastasize.

Under certain conditions, normal cells produce enzymes that break down the tissues that surround them. For example, when tissues are damaged (e.g., because of a wound) cells produce enzymes that destroy the damaged tissues, making way for regrowth. Usually, the cellular systems that produce these destructive enzymes are under very tight control. Occasionally, however, these systems malfunction. For example, one cell within a previously benign growth may mutate and begin to produce enzymes which destroy the membranes and structures that separate the growth from the blood and the lymph. Now the out-of-control cancer cells can leave the site where they were originally growing and can travel (metastasize) to other parts of the body, where they can form secondary tumors. So for a cancer cell to metastasize, mutations must occur which activate control systems that promote growth "in the wrong place." At this point the situation is serious, because although a skilled surgeon can often remove a primary tumor, cancers that have metastasized are frequently fatal.

An important point to take from all of this is that a cell really doesn't need to come up with anything "new" to become a cancer cell. The control systems that must be activated to promote the growth of a cancer cell are normal systems that perform perfectly legitimate, in many cases essential, functions during the life of a cell.

CLASSIFICATION OF CANCER CELLS

Cancer cells can be grouped into two general categories: non-blood-cell cancers (usually referred to as "solid tumors") and blood-cell cancers. Solid tumors are further classified according to the cell type from which they arise. Carcinomas, the most common tumors in humans, are cancers of epithelial cells, and include lung, breast, colon, and cervical cancer, among others. These cancers generally kill by metastasizing to vital organs, where they grow and crowd the organ until it no longer can function properly. Humans also get cancers of the connective and structural tissues, although these "sarcomas" are relatively rare compared to carcinomas. Perhaps the best known example of a sarcoma is bone cancer (osteosarcoma).

Blood-cell cancers make up the other class of human cancers, and the most frequent of these are leukemias and lymphomas. Blood-cell cancers arise when descendants of blood stem cells, which normally should mature into lymphocytes or myeloid cells (e.g., neutrophils), stop maturing and just continue proliferating. In a real sense, these blood cells refuse to "grow up" – and that's the problem. In leukemia, the immature cells fill up the bone marrow and prevent other blood cells from maturing. As a result, the patient usually dies from anemia (due to a scarcity of red blood cells) or from infections (due to a deficit of immune system cells). In lymphoma, large "clusters" of immature cells form in lymph nodes and other secondary lymphoid organs – clusters that in some ways resemble solid tumors. Lymphoma patients usually succumb to infections or organ malfunction.

There is another way to classify human cancers: spontaneous and virus-associated. This classification is especially useful in evaluating the importance of immune surveillance against cancer, because as you will see, immune surveillance is very different in these two cases.

Most human tumors are called spontaneous, because they arise when a single cell accumulates a collection of mutations that causes it to acquire the properties of a cancer cell. These mutations can result from errors made when cellular DNA is copied to be passed down to daughters cells, or from the effects of mutagenic compounds (carcinogens) that are byproducts of normal cellular metabolism or that are present in the air we breathe and the food we eat. Mutations can also be caused by radiation (including UV light) or by errors made in assembling the segments of DNA that make up the B and T cell receptors. As we go through life, these mutations occur "spontaneously," but there are certain factors that can <u>accelerate</u> the rate of mutation: cigarette smoking, a fatty diet, an increased radiation exposure from living at high altitude, working in a plutonium processing plant, etc.

Virus-associated cancers are also "spontaneous" in the sense that mutations caused by errors in DNA copying, carcinogens, and radiation may also be involved. What sets virus-associated cancers apart is that they have, as an additional accelerating factor, a viral infection. For example, essentially all human cervical cancers have, as an accelerating factor, infection by the human papilloma virus. This sexually transmitted virus infects cells that line the uterine cervix, and expresses in these cells viral proteins that can disable two safeguard systems, including the p53 system. Likewise, hepatitis B virus can establish a chronic infection of liver cells, can inactivate p53, and can act as an accelerating factor for liver cancer.

The hallmark of virus-associated cancer is that only a small fraction of infected individuals actually get cancer, yet for those who do, virus or viral genes can usually be recovered from their tumors. For example, less than 1% of the women infected with genital human papilloma virus will ever get cancer of the cervix, yet human papilloma virus genes have been found in over 90% of all cervical carcinomas examined. The reason for this, of course, is that the virus can't cause cancer by itself – it can only accelerate the process that involves the accumulation of cancer-causing mutations.

IMMUNE SURVEILLANCE AGAINST CANCER

From this introduction, it should be clear that powerful defenses exist within the cell (e.g., tumor suppressor proteins) to deal harshly with most wannabe cancer cells. Whether or not the immune system also plays a major role in protecting us against the majority of human cancers is not nearly so clear. There are, of course, many anecdotal (uncontrolled) reports of a connection between the "health" of the immune system and cancer. For example, we have all heard accounts of people who have come down with cancer at times when they were under great stress, and we suppose that stress somehow reduced the strength of their immune systems and allowed a cancer cell to escape immune surveillance. We also have heard stories of patients with "incurable" cancer whose cancers vanished when they changed their diet or began to watch lots of cartoons. We imagine that their new diet or happy thoughts somehow strengthened their immune system, so that it was able to fight off the tumor.

In animals, there is some experimental evidence which suggests that stress can weaken immune defenses against cancer. For example, my friend Jim Cook studies the ability of natural killer cells to kill tumor cells. For many of his studies, he uses natural killer cells that have been "donated" by mice. Jim tells me, however, that when he orders mice to be shipped to him from across the country, he has to let the animals recover for several weeks before he can use their cells. Newly arrived mice are so stressed by the trip that their natural killer cells are not very effective at destroying tumors.

Clearly there is a connection between the human "psyche" and the immune system, but the details of how the mind and the immune system interact have not yet been worked out. Because of this lack of knowledge, it has been impossible so far to identify exact mechanisms by which a person's mental state can influence susceptibility to cancer. In humans whose immune systems have been weakened (immunosuppressed), either by chemotherapy or by diseases such as AIDS, the increased incidence of lymphoma, leukemia, and virus-associated cancer is well documented. However, during immunosuppression, a similar increase is <u>not</u> seen in the most common of all human tumors: spontaneous tumors that are not of blood-cell origin. The same is true with "nude" mice, which are immunodeficient because they lack functional T cells. These mice have an increased incidence of lymphoma and leukemia, but do not get more spontaneous, non-blood cell cancers than normal mice. These results suggest that although immune surveillance may be involved in defending against virus-associated and blood-cell cancers, it probably is not a significant defense against most human tumors.

To try to understand why immune surveillance might be more effective against certain types of cancer than against others, let's examine the roles that various immune system cells may play in surveillance against cancer, keeping in mind that different kinds of cancer may be viewed very differently by these cells.

IMMUNE SURVEILLANCE BY MACROPHAGES AND NK CELLS

Two types of cells that may provide surveillance against some cancers are macrophages and natural killer cells. Hyperactivated macrophages secrete TNF and express it on their surfaces. Either form of TNF can kill certain types of tumor cells in the test tube. This brings up an important point: What happens in the test tube is not always the same as what happens in the animal. For example, there are mouse sarcoma cells that are very resistant to killing by TNF in the test tube. In contrast, when mice that have these same sarcomas are treated with TNF, the tumors are rapidly killed. Studies of this phenomenon showed that the reason TNF is able to kill the tumor when it is in the animal is that this cytokine actually attacks the blood vessels that feed the tumor, cutting off the blood supply, causing the tumor cells to starve to death. This type of death is called "necrosis" and it was this observation that led scientists to name this cytokine "tumor necrosis factor."

In humans, there are examples of cancer therapies in which activated macrophages are likely to play a major role in tumor rejection. One such therapy involves injecting the tumor with BCG, a cousin of the bacterium that causes tuberculosis. BCG hyperactivates macrophages, and when it is injected directly into a tumor (e.g., a melanoma), the tumor fills up with highly activated macrophages that can destroy the cancer. In fact, one of the standard treatments for bladder cancer is injections of BCG – a treatment that is quite effective in eliminating superficial tumors, probably through the action of hyperactivated macrophages.

But how do macrophages tell the difference between normal and cancer cells? The answer to this question is not known for certain, but the evidence suggests that macrophages recognize tumor cells that have unusual cell surface molecules. One of the duties of macrophages in the spleen is to test red blood cells to see if they have become damaged or old. Macrophages use their sense of "feel" to tell which red cells are past their prime, and when they find an old one, they eat it. What macrophages feel for is a fat molecule called phosphatidylserine. This particular fat is usually found on the inside of young red blood cells, but flips to the outside when the cells get old. Like old red blood cells, tumor cells also tend to have unusual surface molecules, and in fact, some express phosphatidylserine on their surfaces. It is believed that the abnormal expression of surface molecules on tumor cells may allow activated macrophages to differentiate between cancer cells and normal cells.

In the test tube, natural killer cells can destroy some tumor cells by using either perforin plus secreted enzymes or Fas ligand to trigger apoptosis. In addition, there is some evidence that NK cells can kill cancer cells in the body. However, these experiments are difficult to interpret, because it is not clear whether NK cells actually do the killing, or whether they simply cooperate by providing cytokines to other cells that kill (e.g., macrophages). Like macrophages, it appears that NK cells select tumor cells for killing because these cells have unusual surface molecules (e.g., proteins that indicate that cancer cells are "stressed").

There would be a number of advantages to having macrophages and NK cells provide surveillance against wannabe cancer cells that look funny on the outside. First, unlike CTLs that take a week or more to get cranked up, macrophages and NK cells are quick-acting. This is an important consideration, because the longer abnormal cells have to proliferate, the higher the likelihood they will mutate to take on the characteristics of metastatic cancer cells. In addition, once a tumor becomes large, it is much more difficult for killer cells to deal with. So you would like the weapons that protect against wannabe cancer cells to be ready to go just as soon as the cells start to get a little weird.

You would also like antitumor weapons to be focused on diverse targets, because a single target (e.g., the MHC-peptide combination seen by a T cell) can be mutated, rendering the target unrecognizable. Both NK cells and macrophages recognize diverse target structures, so the chances of them being fooled by a single mutation is small. Moreover, NK cells and macrophages are located out in the tissues where most tumors arise, so they can intercept cancer cells at an early stage. With immune surveillance, as with real estate, location is everything.

NK cells also have the advantage that they don't need to be activated to kill – the recognition of the correct target structure on a cancer cell seems to be enough. In contrast, macrophages need to be hyperactivated before they can kill cancer cells. So if a wannabe cancer cell arises at a site of inflammation where macrophages are already hyperactivated, that's great. But if there's no inflammatory reaction going on, macrophages will probably remain in a resting state and simply ignore cancer cells. Fortunately, NK cells produce cytokines like IFN-γ that can help activate macrophages. In fact, one of the major functions of NK cells is to provide cytokines to other immune system cells. So if NK cells become irritated due to the presence of cancer cells, they secrete cytokines that can help hyperactivate macrophages – and these hyperactivated macrophages then secrete cytokines (e.g., TNF) that can help hyperactivate NK cells to make them even better killers. This is a good example of the power of "networking" in the immune system.

CTLS AND VIRUS-ASSOCIATED TUMORS

Being infected by certain viruses can predispose a person to contracting particular types of cancer. Because Mother Nature designed killer T cells to defend against viral infections, it is easy to imagine that CTLs might also provide surveillance against virus-associated tumors. Unfortunately, this surveillance is probably quite limited. Here's why.

Cancer arises when multiple cellular control systems are corrupted. In virus-associated cancers, part of this "corruption" results when proteins encoded by the virus interact with control systems within the virus-infected cell. However, the viral infection is only part of the story, because mutations in cellular genes are also required to turn a virus-infected cell into a cancer cell. In a sense, the viral infection "substitutes" for the effect of one or two of the five or so mutations that are required to make a tumor.

Most viruses cause "acute" infections in which, after human cells have been infected and new viruses have been produced, all the virus-infected cells are destroyed and the virus is quickly eradicated by the immune system. Because a dead cell isn't going to make a tumor, viruses that only cause acute infections do not play a role in cancer. This explains why most viral infections are not associated with human cancer.

There are viruses, however, that are able to evade the immune system and establish long-term (sometimes lifelong) infections. Indeed, all viruses which have been shown to play a role in causing cancer are able to establish long-lasting infections by "hiding" from the immune system. It is during this period of hiding that a virus-infected cell accumulates the mutations needed for it to become a full-blown cancer cell. Because CTLs cannot destroy virus-infected cells while they are hiding, and because these hidden cells are the ones that eventually become cancer cells, it can be argued that CTLs do not provide effective surveillance against virus-associated cancer.

Of course, you could postulate that without killer T cells, more cells would be infected during a virus attack, resulting in more virus-infected cells being able to "figure out" how to hide from the immune system. And this is probably true. In fact, this may explain why humans with deficient immune systems have higher than normal rates of virus-associated tumors. However, the bottom line is that although CTLs are great against an acute viral infection, they do not provide significant surveillance against virus-associated cancers, because these cancers only result from long-term viral infections – infections that cannot be detected or cannot be dealt with by CTLs.

CTLS AND SPONTANEOUS TUMORS

So almost by definition, killer T cells do not provide surveillance against virus-infected cells that have become tumor cells. But what about tumors that are not virus-associated? Such tumors make up the majority of human cancers, so perhaps CTLs can provide surveillance against these cancers. Let's evaluate this possibility.

Imagine that a heavy smoker finally accumulates enough mutations in the cells of his lungs to turn one of them into a metastatic tumor cell. Remember, it only takes one bad cell to make a cancer. And let's suppose that because of these mutations, this cell expresses proteins that could be recognized as foreign by Th cells and CTLs. Proteins with this property are usually referred to as "tumor antigens." Now let me ask you a question: Where are the naive T cells while this tumor is growing in the lung? That's right. They are circulating through the blood, lymph, and secondary lymphoid organs. Do they leave this circulation pattern to enter the tissues of the lung? No, not until after they have been activated.

So right away we have a traffic problem. To make self tolerance work, Mother Nature set up the traffic system so that naive T cells don't get out into the tissues where they might encounter self antigens that were not present in the thymus during tolerance induction. As a result, it's unlikely that virgin T cells would ever "see" tumor antigens expressed in the lung – because they just don't go there. What we have here is a serious conflict between the need to preserve tolerance of self (and avoid autoimmune disease) and the need to provide surveillance against tumors that arise, as most tumors do, out in the tissues. And tolerance wins.

Now, sometimes virgin T cells do disobey the traffic laws and wander out into the tissues. So you might imagine that this kind of adventure could give some T cells a chance to look at the tumor that's growing in this guy's lung and be activated. But wait! What is required for T cell activation? First of all, killer T cells must recognize antigens which are produced within a cell and presented by class I MHC molecules on the surface of that cell. This means that the tumor cell itself must do the antigen presentation. But CTLs also require co-stimulation from the cell that presents the antigen. Is this lung tumor cell going to provide that co-stimulation? I don't think so! This isn't an antigen presenting cell, after all. It's a plain old lung cell, and lung cells usually don't express co-stimulatory molecules like B7. Consequently, if a renegade, virgin CTL breaks the traffic laws, enters the lung, and recognizes a tumor antigen, that CTL most likely will be anergized or killed – because the tumor cell cannot provide the co-stimulation the CTL needs for survival.

Again we see a conflict between tolerance induction and tumor surveillance. The two-key system of specific recognition plus co-stimulation was set up so that T cells which recognize self antigens out in the tissues, but which do not receive proper co-stimulation, will be anergized or killed to prevent autoimmunity. Unfortunately, this same two-key system makes it very difficult for CTLs to be activated by tumor cells that arise in the tissues.

Now, you may be thinking that Mother Nature really blew it by designing a system in which tumor surveillance is in conflict with self tolerance. But remember that the main concern in setting up the immune system was to protect us against disease (both microbial and autoimmune) until we are old enough to produce and rear our offspring. Because cancer is mainly a disease that afflicts older persons, surveillance against cancer was not a high priority (i.e., not of selective value) as the immune system evolved.

So the bottom line is that a CTL would have to perform "unnatural acts" to be activated by a tumor out in the tissues: It would have to break the traffic laws and somehow avoid being anergized or killed. This could happen, of course, but it would be very inefficient in comparison to activation of CTLs in response to a viral infection. Alternatively, tumor cells could metastasize to a lymph node, and T cells might be activated there – but by the time this happens, the game is probably over.

The inefficient activation of CTLs by tumor cells is doubly troublesome. If CTLs eventually are activated, they will probably have a large (and perhaps metastatic) tumor to deal with. Even worse, the tumor cells will have had plenty of time to mutate to evade detection by CTLs. Cancer cells mutate like crazy, and there are many different mutations that can prevent recognition or presentation of tumor antigens. For example, the gene encoding the tumor antigen itself can mutate so that the tumor antigen no longer can be recognized by the CTLs, or no longer will fit properly into the groove of an MHC molecule for presentation. In addition, tumor cells can mutate so that they do not produce the MHC molecule that CTLs are restricted to recognize. This happens quite frequently: About 15% of the tumors that have been examined have lost expression of at least one of their MHC molecules. Also, genes that encode the LMP proteins or the TAP transporters can mutate in the tumor cell, with the result that tumor antigens will not be efficiently processed or transported for loading onto class I MHC molecules. This high mutation rate is the tumor's greatest advantage over the immune system, and it usually can keep tumor cells one step ahead of surveillance by CTLs. So even when it occurs, CTL surveillance is most likely a case of "too little, too late."

Okay, so CTLs probably don't provide serious surveillance against non-blood-cell, spontaneous tumors. That's a real bummer, because these make up the majority of human tumors. But what about blood-cell cancers like leukemia and lymphoma? Maybe CTLs are useful against them. After all, immunosuppressed humans and mice do have higher frequencies of leukemia and lymphoma than do normal humans and mice. This suggests that there might be something fundamentally different about the way the immune system views tumors in tissues and organs versus the way it views blood cells that have become cancer cells. Let's take a look at what these differences might be.

One of the difficulties that CTLs have in providing surveillance against tumors that arise in tissues is that these tumors simply are not on the normal traffic pattern of virgin T cells – and it's hard to imagine how a CTL could be activated by an antigen it doesn't see. In contrast, most blood-cell cancers are found in the blood, lymph, and secondary lymphoid organs, and this is ideal for viewing by CTLs, which pass through these areas all the time. Thus, in the case of blood-cell cancers, the traffic patterns of cancer cells and virgin T cells actually intersect. Moreover, in contrast to tumors in tissues, which usually are unable to supply the co-stimulation required for activation of virgin T cells, some cancerous blood cells actually express high levels of B7, and therefore can provide the necessary co-stimulation. These properties of blood-cell cancers suggest that CTLs might provide surveillance against some of them. Unfortunately, this surveillance must be incomplete, because people with otherwise healthy immune systems still get leukemias and lymphomas.

My conclusion is that CTLs, by their nature, are not very good at providing surveillance against cancer cells. Nevertheless, immunologists have shown that CTLs from some cancer patients can kill tumor cells in the test tube. On the basis of these findings, immunologists hope that CTLs or tumor cells can be manipulated so that CTLs will learn to kill tumor cells efficiently in the patient. Early evidence suggests that in a few cases this may be possible, although the realistic goal of this approach is to treat the "minimum residual disease" that remains after a surgeon has removed the primary tumor. Of course, we can all hope that these experiments will be successful, because about a third of us will get cancer during our lifetimes. Nevertheless, until immu-nologists learn to "trick" our immune systems into destroying tumors, we'd better eat right, be careful what we take into our lungs, and stay out of the sun!

THOUGHT QUESTIONS

1. Why must multiple control systems be corrupted before a cell becomes a cancer cell?

2. There are two ways that cellular control systems can be corrupted, leading to cancer. What are they?

3. Why is cancer primarily a disease that affects older people?

4. Some human cancers are said to be "virus-associated." What does this mean?

5. Is there a conflict between immune surveillance against cancer and the preservation of tolerance to self antigens? Explain.

6. Explain why the adaptive immune system may provide effective surveillance against blood-cell cancers, but not against spontaneous, non-blood-cell cancers.

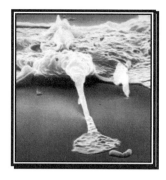

GLOSSARY

ADCC   Antibody-dependent cellular cytotoxicity. Antibodies bind to the target, and Fc receptors on the surfaces of cytotoxic cells (e.g., macrophages and NK cells) bind to the antibodies to form a "bridge" between the target and the cytotoxic cell: antibody-directed killing.

Allergen   An antigen that causes allergies.

Anergy   A state of non-functionality.

Antigen   A rather loosely used term for the target (e.g., a viral protein) of an antibody or a T cell. To be more precise, an antibody binds to a <u>region</u> of an antigen called the epitope, and the T cell receptor binds to a peptide that is a <u>fragment</u> of the antigen.

Anti-oncogene   A gene that encodes a tumor suppressor protein.

APC   Antigen presenting cell – cells like activated macrophages, dendritic cells, and B cells that can present antigen efficiently to T cells via MHC molecules, and which can supply the co-stimulatory molecules required to activate T cells.

Apoptosis   Sometimes called programmed cell death. The process by which cells commit suicide in response to problems within the cell or signals from outside the cell.

Autocrine   A fancy word for "self" (e.g., autocrine stimulation is self stimulation).

BCR   B cell receptor.

β2-microglobulin   The non-polymorphic chain of the class I MHC molecule.

Central tolerance induction   Process by which T cells with receptors that recognize abundant self antigens in the thymus are anergized or deleted.

Chemokine   A type of cytokine which helps direct the trafficking of immune system cells by acting as a chemoattractant.

Clonal selection principle   When receptors on B or T cells recognize their cognate antigen, these cells are triggered (selected) to proliferate. As a result, a clone of B or T cells with identical antigen specificities is produced.

Cognate antigen   The antigen (e.g., a bacterial protein) that a B or T cell's receptors recognize and bind to.

Co-receptor   The CD4 or CD8 molecule on T cells, or the complement receptor on B cells.

Co-stimulation   The second "key" that B and T cells need for activation.

Crosslink   Cluster together (e.g., an antigen may crosslink B cell receptors).

Cross reacts   Recognizes several different epitopes. For example, a B cell's receptors may bind to (cross react with) several different epitopes that are present on several different antigens.

CTL   Cytotoxic lymphocyte – synonym for killer T cell.

Cytokines   Hormone-like messenger molecules that cells use to communicate.

Cytokine profile   The mixture of different cytokines that a cell secretes.

Cytoplasm   The liquid portion of a cell in which the organelles and the nucleus "float."

DC   Dendritic cell – a starfish-shaped cell that functions as an antigen presenting cell for T cells.

DTH   Delayed type hypersensitivity. An inflammatory reaction in which Th cells recognize a specific invader, and secrete cytokines that activate and recruit innate system cells to do the killing.

Endocytosis   Similar to phagocytosis except that it begins when the thing being "eaten" binds to a receptor on the surface of the phagocytic cell: receptor-initiated phagocytosis.

Endogenous protein   A protein that is produced within the cell in question – the opposite of an exogenous protein.

Endoplasmic reticulum   A large sack-like structure inside the cell from which most proteins destined for transport to the cell surface begin their journey.

Endothelial cells   Cells shaped like shingles that line the insides of our blood vessels.

Epithelial cells   Cells that form part of the barrier that separates our bodies from the outside world.

Epitope   The region of an antigen that is recognized by a B or T cell's receptors.

Exogenous protein   A protein that is outside the cell in question – the opposite of an endogenous protein.

FDC   Follicular dendritic cell – a starfish-shaped cell that retains opsonized antigens in germinal centers and displays these antigens for B cells to see.

Germinal center   An area in a secondary lymphoid organ in which B cells proliferate, undergo somatic hypermutation, and switch classes. Also known as a "secondary lymphoid follicle."

Hc   Heavy chain protein of the antibody molecule.

High endothelial venule (HEV)   A region in a blood vessel where there are high endothelial cells that allow lymphocytes to exit the blood.

IFN-γ   Interferon gamma – a cytokine secreted mainly by Th1 helper T cells and NK cells.

Inflammatory response   A rather general term that describes the battle that macrophages, neutrophils, and other immune system cells wage against an invader.

Interleukin   A protein (cytokine) that is used for communication between leukocytes (e.g., IL-2).

Isotype   A synonym for "class." The isotype of an antibody (e.g., IgA or IgG) is determined by the constant region of its heavy chain.

Lc   Light chain protein of the antibody molecule.

Leukocytes   A generic term that includes all of the different kinds of white blood cells.

Ligand   A molecule that binds to a receptor (e.g., the Fas ligand binds to the Fas receptor protein on the surface of a cell).

Ligate   Bind to. When a receptor has bound its ligand, it is said to be "ligated."

Lymph   The liquid that "leaks" out of blood vessels into the tissues.

Lymphocytes   B cells and T cells.

Lymphoid follicle   A region of a secondary lymphoid organ that contains follicular dendritic cells embedded in a sea of B cells.

M cell   A cell that crowns a Peyer's patch, and which specializes in sampling antigen from the intestine.

MALT   Mucosal associated lymphoid tissues. Secondary lymphoid organs that are associated with mucosa (e.g., Peyers patches and tonsils).

MHC proteins   Proteins encoded by the major histocompatibility complex (the region of a chromosome that includes a "complex" of genes involved in antigen presentation).

MHC restriction   Survival in the thymus is "restricted" to T cells whose receptors recognize antigen presented by MHC molecules.

Microbe   A generic term that includes bacteria and viruses.

Monocytes   White blood cells that are the precursors of macrophages and dendritic cells.

Mucosa   The tissues and associated mucus that protect exposed surfaces such as the gastrointestinal and respiratory tracts.

Necrosis   Cell death, typically caused by burns or other trauma. This type of cell death (as opposed to apoptotic cell death) usually results in the contents of the cell being dumped into the tissues where it can cause damage.

Negative selection   Synonym for "central tolerance induction."

NK cell   Natural killer cell – a player on the innate system team.

Oncogene   A mutated proto-oncogene which encodes a protein that can cause cells to proliferate inappropriately.

Opsonize   "Decorate" with fragments of complement proteins or with antibodies.

Pathogen   A disease-causing agent (e.g., a bacterium or a virus).

Peptide   A small fragment of a protein, usually only tens of amino acids in length.

Peripheral tolerance   The mechanisms that induce self tolerance outside the thymus.

Phagocytes   Cells like macrophages and neutrophils that engulf (phagocytose) invaders.

Positive selection   Synonym for "MHC restriction."

Primary lymphoid organs The thymus and the bone marrow.

Proliferate Increase in number. A cell proliferates by dividing into two daughter cells, which then can divide again to give four cells, and so on.

Proteasome A multi-protein complex in the cell that chops proteins up into small pieces.

Proto-oncogene A gene which, if mutated, can become an oncogene.

Secondary lymphoid organs Organs like the lymph nodes, Peyer's patches, and the spleen where activation of naive B and T cells takes place.

Secrete Export out of the cell (e.g., cytokines are secreted by the T cells that produce them).

TCR T cell receptor.

Th Helper T cell.

TNF Tumor necrosis factor – a cytokine secreted mainly by macrophages and helper T cells.

Tumor suppressor protein A protein which is part of a control system within a cell that safeguards against inappropriate cell proliferation.

Virgin (naive) lymphocytes B and T cells that have never been activated.

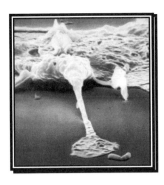

INDEX

natural killer cell activity in, 22–23, 24
autoimmune disease and, 102
rheumatoid arthritis and, 103
sepsis and, 98
Tumors. *See* Cancer
Tumor suppressor genes, 109–110
Tumor suppressor protein, 109, 119

U

Uterus, 56

V

Vaccinations, 6
Venules, high endothelial, 74–75, 77–78, 83, 118
V gene segment, 7, 28–29, 38
Viruses, 40
    acute infection, 105, 114
    adaptive immune system and, 5
    antibody response to, 8, 37–38

autoimmune disease and, 101
cancer associated with, 110, 111–112, 114
    cytotoxic lymphocytes in, 113–114
chronic, 105–106
cytotoxic lymphocytes, 66
    in cancer, 113–114
    in HIV infection, 105–106
expression of MHC molecules and, 35
in HIV infection, 105–106
innate immune system and, 24
    natural killer cell activation in, 22–23
interferon response to, 18
latent infection, 106
opsonization of, 8
tumor necrosis factor and, 19
vaccination against, 6
Virgin lymphocytes, 119

Z

ζ protein, 57